Hormones

Recent Titles in
Q&A Health Guides

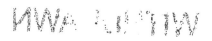

HORMONES

❖

Your Questions Answered

Tish Davidson

Q&A Health Guides

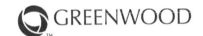
GREENWOOD
An Imprint of ABC-CLIO, LLC
Santa Barbara, California • Denver, Colorado

This book discusses treatments (including types of medication and mental health therapies), diagnostic tests for various symptoms and mental health disorders, and organizations. The authors have made every effort to present accurate and up-to-date information. However, the information in this book is not intended to recommend or endorse particular treatments or organizations, or substitute for the care or medical advice of a qualified health professional, or used to alter any medical therapy without a medical doctor's advice. Specific situations may require specific therapeutic approaches not included in this book. For those reasons, we recommend that readers follow the advice of qualified health care professionals directly involved in their care. Readers who suspect they may have specific medical problems should consult a physician about any suggestions made in this book.

Library of Congress Cataloging-in-Publication Data

Names: Davidson, Tish, author.
Title: Hormones : your questions answered / Tish Davidson.
Description: Santa Barbara, California : Greenwood, an Imprint of ABC-CLIO,
   LLC, [2022] | Series: Q&A health guides | Includes bibliographical
   references and index.
Identifiers: LCCN 2022012570 | ISBN 9781440877315 (hardcover) | ISBN
   9781440877322 (ebook)
Subjects: LCSH: Hormones. | Hormones—Miscellanea.
Classification: LCC QP571 .D38 2022 | DDC 612.4/05—dc23/eng/20220401
LC record available at https://lccn.loc.gov/2022012570

ISBN: 978-1-4408-7731-5 (print)
         978-1-4408-7732-2 (ebook)

26 25 24 23 22   1 2 3 4 5

This book is also available as an eBook.

Greenwood
An Imprint of ABC-CLIO, LLC

ABC-CLIO, LLC
147 Castilian Drive
Santa Barbara, California 93117
www.abc-clio.com

This book is printed on acid-free paper ∞

Manufactured in the United States of America

Contents

Series Foreword

All of us have questions about our health. Is this normal? Should I be doing something differently? Whom should I talk to about my concerns? And our modern world is full of answers. Thanks to the Internet, there's a wealth of information at our fingertips, from forums where people can share their personal experiences to Wikipedia articles to the full text of medical studies. But finding the right information can be an intimidating and difficult task—some sources are written at too high a level, others have been oversimplified, while still others are heavily biased or simply inaccurate.

Q&A Health Guides address the needs of readers who want accurate, concise answers to their health questions, authored by reputable and objective experts, and written in clear and easy-to-understand language. This series focuses on the topics that matter most to young adult readers, including various aspects of physical and emotional well-being as well as other components of a healthy lifestyle. These guides will also serve as a valuable tool for parents, school counselors, and others who may need to answer teens' health questions.

All books in the series follow the same format to make finding information quick and easy. Each volume begins with an essay on health literacy and why it is so important when it comes to gathering and evaluating health information. Next, the top five myths and misconceptions that surround the topic are dispelled. The heart of each guide is a collection of questions and answers, organized thematically. A selection of five case studies provides real-world examples to illuminate key concepts. Rounding out each volume are a directory of resources, glossary, and index.

It is our hope that the books in this series will not only provide valuable information but will also help guide readers toward a lifetime of healthy decision making.

Acknowledgments

Writing a book is a long, challenging, and essentially solitary process but especially so during the COVID-19 pandemic. This book came into existence because of the support of some outstanding and dedicated people. It could not have been written without the librarians of the Alameda County Library System who worked patiently to acquire needed reference material from libraries across the West despite pandemic shutdowns. Thanks also to my gifted editor, Maxine Taylor. Her thoughtful suggestions and editorial guidance helped shape this book into what it is today. Scott Davidson and Helen Colby deserve a special mention for taking time to give feedback on the manuscript when COVID-19 disrupted my regular critique group. Finally, appreciation goes to the production team at ABC-CLIO. It always surprises me how they can work their magic and turn pages and pages of black-and-white manuscript into an attractive, accessible book.

Introduction

Learning about hormones is a bit like doing a jigsaw puzzle without a picture on the box. You can see all the individual pieces, but you can't figure out the whole picture until you put most of the pieces together. It is the same with hormones. You can understand the origin and actions of each individual hormone, but it is hard to get an accurate picture of how they work together in the body until you understand something about many of them. In addition, hormones interact with each other as well as with target tissues. Sorting out these interactions may at first feel like trying to use a transportation map of New York City with local and express subway lines, busses, and ferries going to all five boroughs and intersecting with each other at multiple points.

The idea of hormones—signaling molecules that travel through the bloodstream in tiny quantities and change the activity of tissues distant from their source—did not take off until the early 1900s. Because hormones could not be seen or measured, before that most scientists believed all signaling occurred through nerves. The real breakthrough in hormone research came in 1921, when a team of Canadian scientists isolated insulin, a hormone that regulates blood sugar levels. Since that time, the lives of millions of people with diabetes who lack the ability to produce insulin have been saved. The success of insulin—and the Nobel Prize that went to its discoverers—increased interest in hormones. Still, a major hurdle remained. Hormones are secreted in such tiny quantities that it took until 1959 to develop a way to accurately measure them in the blood.

In the 2020s, new hormones are still being discovered, and new discoveries are being made about familiar hormones. For example, scientists have discovered that men make prolactin, a hormone that causes women to make breast milk. Why? What does prolactin do in men? That question remains to be answered. Other researchers are studying how certain hormones interact with common substances such as caffeine, alcohol, marijuana, and artificial sweeteners and even how they affect risk-taking.

This book explores the mechanisms by which hormones regulate basic body functions, how they affect behavior, and how human activities affect them. The book is arranged in question-and-answer form to help simplify explanations of the way hormones work together to keep the body in balance, and running smoothly, and to show what happens when interruptions in the hormonal communication system occur. After reading some of the basics, the questions can be read in any order.

Guide to Health Literacy

On her 13th birthday, Samantha was diagnosed with type 2 diabetes. She consulted her mom and her aunt, both of whom also have type 2 diabetes, and decided to go with their strategy of managing diabetes by taking insulin. As a result of participating in an after-school program at her middle school that focused on health literacy, she learned that she can help manage the level of glucose in her bloodstream by counting her carbohydrate intake, following a diabetic diet, and exercising regularly. But, what exactly should she do? How does she keep track of her carbohydrate intake? What is a diabetic diet? How long should she exercise and what type of exercise should she do? Samantha is a visual learner, so she turned to her favorite source of media, YouTube, to answer these questions. She found videos from individuals around the world sharing their experiences and tips, doctors (or at least people who have "Dr." in their YouTube channel names), government agencies such as the National Institutes of Health, and even video clips from cat lovers who have cats with diabetes. With guidance from the librarian and the health and science teachers at her school, she assessed the credibility of the information in these videos and even compared their suggestions to some of the print resources that she was able to find at her school library. Now, she knows exactly how to count her carbohydrate level, how to prepare and follow a diabetic diet, and how much (and what) exercise is needed daily. She intends to share her findings with her mom and her aunt, and now she wants to create a chart that summarizes what she has learned that she can share with her doctor.

Samantha's experience is not unique. She represents a shift in our society; an individual no longer views himself or herself as a passive recipient of medical care but as an active mediator of his or her own health. However, in this era when any individual can post his or her opinions and experiences with a particular health condition online with just a few clicks or publish a memoir, it is vital that people know how to assess the credibility of health information. Gone are the days when "publishing" health information required intense vetting. The health information landscape is highly saturated, and people have innumerable sources where they can find information about practically any health topic. The sources (whether print, online, or a person) that an individual consults for health information are crucial because the accuracy and trustworthiness of the information can potentially affect his or her overall health. The ability to find, select, assess, and use health information constitutes a type of literacy—health literacy—that everyone must possess.

THE DEFINITION AND PHASES OF HEALTH LITERACY

One of the most popular definitions for health literacy comes from Ratzan and Parker (2000), who describe health literacy as "the degree to which individuals have the capacity to obtain, process, and understand basic health information and services needed to make appropriate health decisions." Recent research has extrapolated health literacy into health literacy bits, further shedding light on the multiple phases and literacy practices that are embedded within the multifaceted concept of health literacy. Although this research has focused primarily on online health information seeking, these health literacy bits are needed to successfully navigate both print and online sources. There are six phases of health information seeking: (1) Information Need Identification and Question Formulation, (2) Information Search, (3) Information Comprehension, (4) Information Assessment, (5) Information Management, and (6) Information Use.

The first phase is the *information need identification and question formulation phase*. In this phase, one needs to be able to develop and refine a range of questions to frame one's search and understand relevant health terms. In the second phase, *information search*, one has to possess appropriate searching skills, such as using proper keywords and correct spelling in search terms, especially when using search engines and databases. It is also crucial to understand how search engines work (i.e., how search results are derived, what the order of the search results means, how to use the snippets that are provided in the search results list to select websites, and how to determine which listings are ads on a search engine results page). One also has to limit reliance on surface characteristics, such as the design of a website or a book (a website or book that appears to have a lot of information or looks aesthetically pleasant does not necessarily mean it has good information) and language used (a website or book that utilizes jargon, the keywords that one used to conduct the search, or the word "information" does not necessarily indicate it will have good information). The next phase is *information comprehension*, whereby one needs to have the ability to read, comprehend, and recall the information (including textual, numerical, and visual content) one has located from the books and/or online resources.

To assess the credibility of health information (*information assessment* phase), one needs to be able to evaluate information for accuracy, evaluate how current the information is (e.g., when a website was last updated or when a book was published), and evaluate the creators of the source—for example, examine site sponsors or type of sites (.com, .gov, .edu, or .org) or the author of a book (practicing doctor, a celebrity doctor, a patient of a specific disease, etc.) to determine the believability of the person/ organization providing the information. Such credibility perceptions tend to become generalized, so they must be frequently reexamined (e.g., the belief that a specific news agency always has credible health information needs continuous vetting). One also needs to evaluate the credibility of the medium (e.g., television, Internet, radio, social media, and book) and evaluate—not just accept without questioning—others' claims regarding the validity of a site, book, or other specific source of information. At this stage, one has to "make sense of information gathered from diverse sources by identifying misconceptions, main and supporting ideas, con-flicting information, point of view, and biases" (American Association of School Librarians [AASL], 2009, p. 13) and conclude which sources/ information are valid and accurate by using conscious strategies rather than simply using intuitive judgments or "rules of thumb." This phase is the most challenging segment of health information seeking and serves as a determinant of success (or lack thereof) in the information-seeking process. The following section on Sources of Health Information further explains this phase.

The fifth phase is *information management*, whereby one has to organize information that has been gathered in some manner to ensure easy retrieval and use in the future. The last phase is *information use*, in which one will synthesize information found across various resources, draw conclusions, and locate the answer to his or her original question and/ or the content that fulfills the information need. This phase also often involves implementation, such as using the information to solve a health problem; make health-related decisions; identify and engage in behaviors that will help a person to avoid health risks; share the health information found with family members and friends who may benefit from it; and advocate more broadly for personal, family, or community health.

THE IMPORTANCE OF HEALTH LITERACY

The conception of health has moved from a passive view (someone is either well or ill) to one that is more active and process based (someone is working toward preventing or managing disease). Hence, the dominant focus has shifted from doctors and treatments to patients and prevention, resulting in the need to strengthen our ability and confidence (as patients and consumers of health care) to look for, assess, understand, manage, share, adapt, and use health-related information. An individual's health literacy level has been found to predict his or her health status better than age, race, educational attainment, employment status, and income level (National Network of Libraries of Medicine, 2013). Greater health literacy also enables individuals to better communicate with health care providers such as doctors, nutritionists, and therapists, as they can pose more relevant, informed, and useful questions to health care providers. Another added advantage of greater health literacy is better information-seeking skills, not only for health but also in other domains, such as completing assignments for school.

SOURCES OF HEALTH INFORMATION: THE GOOD, THE BAD, AND THE IN-BETWEEN

For generations, doctors, nurses, nutritionists, health coaches, and other health professionals have been the trusted sources of health information. Additionally, researchers have found that young adults, when they have health-related questions, typically turn to a family member who has had firsthand experience with a health condition because of their family member's close proximity and because of their past experience with, and trust in, this individual. Expertise should be a core consideration when consulting a person, website, or book for health information. The credentials and background of the person or author and conflicting interests of the author (and his or her organization) must be checked and validated to ensure the likely credibility of the health information they are conveying. While books often have implied credibility because of the peer-review process involved, self-publishing has challenged this credibility, so qualifications of book authors should also be verified. When it comes to health information, currency of the source must also be examined. When examining health information/studies presented, pay attention to the exhaustiveness of research methods utilized to offer recommendations or conclusions. Small and nondiverse sample size is often—but not always—an indication of reduced credibility. Studies that confuse correlation with causation is another potential issue to watch for. Information seekers must also pay attention to the sponsors of the research studies. For example, if a study is sponsored by manufacturers of drug Y and the study recommends that drug Y is the best treatment to manage or cure a disease, this may indicate a lack of objectivity on the part of the researchers.

The Internet is rapidly becoming one of the main sources of health information. Online forums, news agencies, personal blogs, social media sites, pharmacy sites, and celebrity "doctors" are all offering medical and health information targeted to various types of people in regard to all types of diseases and symptoms. There are professional journalists, citizen journalists, hoaxers, and people paid to write fake health news on various sites that may appear to have a legitimate domain name and may even have authors who claim to have professional credentials, such as an MD. All these sites *may* offer useful information or information that appears to be useful and relevant; however, much of the information may be debatable and may fall into gray areas that require readers to discern credibility, reliability, and biases.

While broad recognition and acceptance of certain media, institutions, and people often serve as the most popular determining factors to assess credibility of health information among young people, keep in mind that there are legitimate Internet sites, databases, and books that publish health information and serve as sources of health information for doctors, other health sites, and members of the public. For example, MedlinePlus (https://medlineplus.gov) has trusted sources on over 975 diseases and conditions and presents the information in easy-to-understand language.

The chart here presents factors to consider when assessing credibility of health information. However, keep in mind that these factors function only as a guide and require continuous updating to keep abreast with the changes in the landscape of health information, information sources, and technologies.

The chart can serve as a guide; however, approaching a librarian about how one can go about assessing the credibility of both print and online health information is far more effective than using generic checklist-type

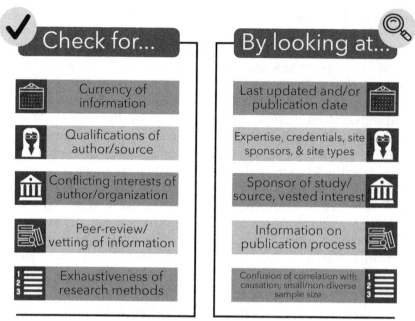

All images from flaticon.com

tools. While librarians are not health experts, they can apply and teach patrons strategies to determine the credibility of health information.

With the prevalence of fake sites and fake resources that appear to be legitimate, it is important to use the following health information assessment tips to verify health information that one has obtained (St. Jean et al., 2015, p. 151):

- **Don't assume you are right**: Even when you feel very sure about an answer, keep in mind that the answer may not be correct, and it is important to conduct (further) searches to validate the information.
- **Don't assume you are wrong**: You may actually have correct information, even if the information you encounter does not match—that is, you may be right and the resources that you have found may contain false information.
- **Take an open approach**: Maintain a critical stance by not including your preexisting beliefs as keywords (or letting them influence your choice of keywords) in a search, as this may influence what it is possible to find out.
- **Verify, verify, and verify**: Information found, especially on the Internet, needs to be validated, no matter how the information appears on

the site (i.e., regardless of the appearance of the site or the quantity of information that is included).

Health literacy comes with experience navigating health information. Professional sources of health information, such as doctors, health care providers, and health databases, are still the best, but one also has the power to search for health information and then verify it by consulting with these trusted sources and by using the health information assessment tips and guide shared previously.

Mega Subramaniam, PhD
Associate Professor, College of Information Studies,
University of Maryland

REFERENCES AND FURTHER READING

American Association of School Librarians (AASL). (2009). *Standards for the 21st-century learner in action.* Chicago, IL: American Association of School Librarians.

Hilligoss, B., & Rieh, S.-Y. (2008). Developing a unifying framework of credibility assessment: Construct, heuristics, and interaction in context. *Information Processing & Management, 44*(4), 1467–1484.

Kuhlthau, C. C. (1988). Developing a model of the library search process: Cognitive and affective aspects. *Reference Quarterly, 28*(2), 232–242.

National Network of Libraries of Medicine (NNLM). (2013). *Health literacy.* Bethesda, MD: National Network of Libraries of Medicine. Retrieved from nnlm.gov/outreach/consumer/hlthlit.html

Ratzan, S. C., & Parker, R. M. (2000). Introduction. In C. R. Selden, M. Zorn, S. C. Ratzan, & R. M. Parker (Eds.), *National Library of Medicine current bibliographies in medicine: Health literacy.* NLM Pub. No. CBM 2000–1. Bethesda, MD: National Institutes of Health, U.S. Department of Health and Human Services.

St. Jean, B., Taylor, N. G., Kodama, C., & Subramaniam, M. (February 2017). Assessing the health information source perceptions of tweens using card-sorting exercises. *Journal of Information Science.* Retrieved from http://journals.sagepub.com/doi/abs/10.1177/0165551516687728

St. Jean, B., Subramaniam, M., Taylor, N. G., Follman, R., Kodama, C., & Casciotti, D. (2015). The influence of positive hypothesis testing on youths' online health-related information seeking. *New Library World, 116*(3/4), 136–154.

Subramaniam, M., St. Jean, B., Taylor, N. G., Kodama, C., Follman, R., & Casciotti, D. (2015). Bit by bit: Using design-based research to improve the health literacy of adolescents. *JMIR Research Protocols*, 4(2), paper e62. Retrieved from http://www.ncbi.nlm.nih.gov/pmc /articles/PMC4464334/

Valenza, J. (2016, November 26). Truth, truthiness, and triangulation: A news literacy toolkit for a "post-truth" world [Web log]. Retrieved from http://blogs.slj.com/neverendingsearch/2016/11/26/truth-truthiness -triangulation-and-the-librarian-way-a-news-literacy-toolkit-for -a-post-truth-world/

Common Misconceptions about Hormones

1. MEN AND WOMEN MAKE DIFFERENT HORMONES

Testosterone is associated with men and estrogen with women, but women also make testosterone, and men make estrogen. The difference is in the quantity of each hormone they make. Both hormones are essential to the health of either sex. Men and women also both make oxytocin and prolactin, hormones associated with giving birth and producing breast milk. Why do men make these hormones? Researchers are not sure about what prolactin does in men, but they think they know why men make oxytocin. For more, see question 6.

2. PREMENSTRUAL SYNDROME (PMS) IS NOT A REAL DISORDER

The physical, emotional, and behavioral symptoms of premenstrual syndrome are real, although not every woman experiences them. The symptoms range from mildly annoying to so severe as to interfere with daily life. About three-quarters of all women are affected by premenstrual symptoms at some point during their reproductive years. What causes premenstrual syndrome? See question 16.

3. SEX IS DETERMINED BY GENETICS, BUT GENDER IDENTITY IS A CHOICE

A person's sex is determined at conception by chromosomes inherited from their parents. Males have XY chromosomes, and females are XX. Gender identity is a deeply held internal belief by individuals about their gender. Sometimes gender identity does not match the individual's inherited chromosomes. There is debate over why some people's gender identity is different from their biological sex. Researchers believe this could be caused by the actions of fetal hormones during development and the effects the hormones have on the organization of the fetal brain. For the implications of this, see question 26.

4. TEENS CHOOSE TO STAY UP LATE TO KEEP UP WITH SCHOOLWORK AND ONLINE SOCIAL LIFE

Teens tend to go to bed much later than when they were younger. This means they get less sleep than experts believe they need. Some of these late hours are due to heavy homework loads and active social media lives, but nature is also working against teens going to bed early. The secretion pattern of the hormone melatonin shifts during the teenage years, making it harder to fall asleep early. For more, see question 32.

5. CONSUMING CAFFEINE HAS NO EFFECT ON HORMONES

Caffeine is the most commonly consumed drug on the planet. It can temporarily heighten alertness, increase blood pressure, and alter mood. How? Drinking coffee, a caffeinated soda, or an energy drink stimulates the release of some of the same hormones that prepare the body for a flight or fight when faced with situations that cause fear or anxiety. For more, see question 42.

Table of Major Hormones

Hormone	Abbreviation	Produced by	Main Functions
Adrenocortico-tropic hormone	ACTH	Anterior pituitary	Stimulates the adrenals to pro-duce cortisol
Aldosterone	None	Adrenal cortex	Regulates blood pressure, sodium, and fluid balance
Antidiuretic hormone (vasopressin)	ADH	Hypothalamus, but stored and released by posterior pituitary	Regulates fluid balance by con-trolling water reabsorption by kidneys
Calcitonin	None	C-cells embed-ded in the thyroid	Reduces calcium levels in blood
Corticotropin-releasing hormone	CRH	Hypothalamus	Stimulates the production of adrenocortico-tropic hormone

(Continued)

Hormone	Abbreviation	Produced by	Main Functions
Cortisol	None	Adrenal cortex	Regulates blood pressure; suppresses inflammation
Dehydroepi-androsterone	DHEA	Adrenal cortex	Converted to testosterone in males and estrogen in females
Epinephrine (adrenaline)	None	Adrenal medulla	Increases heart rate and blood flow; prepares body for action
Estrogen (oestrogen)	E1, E2, E3	Ovaries and also the placenta during pregnancy	Promotes female sexual characteristics and regulates female reproductive system
Follicle-stimulating hormone	FSH	Anterior pituitary	Women: maturation of egg in follicle of ovary before ovulation; men: production of sperm
Ghrelin	None	Stomach	Stimulates sensation of hunger
Glucagon	None	Pancreas	Raises blood glucose levels
Gonadotropin-releasing hormone	GnRH	Hypothalamus	Stimulates production of follicle-stimulating hormone and luteinizing hormone
Growth hormone (somatotropin)	GH, hGH	Anterior pituitary	Stimulates protein synthesis and growth

(Continued)

Hormone	Abbreviation	Produced by	Main Functions
Growth hormone-inhibiting hormone (somatostatin)	GHIH	Hypothalamus	Prevents the anterior pituitary from making growth hormone
Growth hormone-releasing hormone	GHRH	Hypothalamus	Stimulates release of growth hormone
Human chorionic gonadotropin	hCG	Placenta	Causes production of progesterone to support pregnancy
Insulin	None	Pancreas	Lowers blood glucose levels
Leptin	None	Fat cells	Helps to inhibit hunger and regulates long-term energy balance
Luteinizing hormone	LH	Anterior pituitary	Women: stimulates ovary to produce estrogen and release mature egg; men: stimulates production of testosterone
Melatonin	None	Pineal	Helps to regulate sleep-wake cycle
Norepinephrine (noradrenaline)	None	Adrenal medulla	Increases heart rate and blood pressure to prepare body for action
Oxytocin	None	Hypothalamus, but stored and released by posterior pituitary	Stimulates contractions during childbirth; social bonding

(Continued)

Hormone	Abbreviation	Produced by	Main Functions
Parathyroid hormone	PTH	Parathyroid glands	Increases calcium concentration in blood
Progesterone	None	Corpus luteum during menstrual cycle and placenta during pregnancy	Prepares placenta for implantation and maintains pregnancy
Prolactin (lactotropin)	None	Anterior pituitary	Stimulates production of breast milk in nursing women
Relaxin	None	Women: corpus luteum and placenta; men: prostate gland	Women: inhibits uterine contractions; softens cervix before birth; men: increases sperm motility
Testosterone	None	Testes	Matures and maintains male reproductive system functions
Thyroid hormone	T3, T4	Thyroid	Regulates cellular metabolism
Thyroid-stimulating hormone	TSH	Anterior pituitary	Stimulates production and release of thyroid hormone
Thyrotropin-releasing hormone	TRH	Hypothalamus	Stimulates production of thyroid-stimulating hormone

QUESTIONS AND ANSWERS

❖❖❖

The Basics

1. What are hormones?

Hormones are regulatory chemicals made and secreted by tissues in one part of the body and carried by the circulatory system to distant tissues where they have an effect only on specific target cells. The word "hormone" comes from a Greek word meaning "to stimulate" or "to set in motion." In short, a hormone is a chemical signal that stimulates activity in other cells located at a distance from the place where the hormone is produced.

Tissues that make hormones are called endocrine glands. Endocrine glands are ductless glands—that is, they release hormones directly into the bloodstream. This makes them different from other familiar glands such as sweat glands or salivary glands (called exocrine glands) whose products move through ducts (tubules) to a specific location where they are released. Although the collection of hormone-secreting glands is called the endocrine system, the glands of the endocrine system are not physically connected to each other the way other body systems such as the digestive or nervous system are connected.

All multicellular organisms—even plants and fungi—make hormones. Some plant hormones, for example, determine which cells become roots and which become shoots, while others cause the plant to lean in the direction of sunlight. In humans, hormones regulate growth, initiate puberty, control the reproductive cycle, regulate fluid balance, control the use of glucose (sugar) for energy, affect sleep cycles and mood swings, activate the body for flight or fight, promote bonding between mother and child, and stimulate or repress hunger. Hormones are effective in extremely small quantities (parts per billion in the blood). Production of too little or too much of a hormone or failure of the target tissue to respond to the hormone will cause health disorders, some of which can be fatal.

The major endocrine glands have been known to scientists and physicians for many years. However, researchers only recently found that individual cells in the lining of the digestive system and elsewhere can secrete hormones. They have also learned that the same hormone may be produced in more than one place in the body. These discoveries open up new areas of research such as how hormones are related to other signaling molecules. Neuroendocrinologists, for example, are studying the interaction between the nervous system and the endocrine system and how the brain regulates hormonal activity. Behavioral endocrinologists are exploring the effects of hormones on behavior, mood, and emotional responses.

2. How is the endocrine system organized?

The hypothalamus is the master switchboard for the endocrine system. It is an almond-sized organ located on the underside of the brain near the brain stem. Above it is the thalamus, a part of the brain that relays sensory and motor information to other parts of the brain. Below and attached to the hypothalamus by a thin stalk of tissue lies the pituitary gland.

Although the hypothalamus is part of the brain, it contains both nerve and endocrine cells. This allows it to receive information from both the nervous system and from its own embedded sensors that monitor the composition of blood and the concentration of circulating hormones. Together this continuous monitoring allows the hypothalamus to direct the production of hormones that control body temperature, heart rate, thirst, hunger, and fluid balance. It also regulates many aspects of sexual behavior; mother-child bonding; and the body's response to danger, emotions, and stress.

The hypothalamus affects so many body functions by producing releasing hormones. Releasing hormones are hormones that signal the anterior lobe of the pituitary to make or inhibit the making of other hormones that are then secreted into the bloodstream. The hypothalamus produces seven major releasing hormones. Five of them stimulate the production of other hormones, and two inhibit the production of specific hormones. These hormones affect every aspect of metabolism and reproduction. They are listed in the Table of Major Hormones. The hypothalamus also makes two other hormones—antidiuretic hormone (ADH, also called vasopressin) and oxytocin—that are transported from the hypothalamus to the posterior lobe of the pituitary and are released by the pituitary.

The **pituitary** gland is a piece of endocrine tissue about the size of a pea dangling off the hypothalamus. It is divided into two parts: the anterior lobe and the posterior lobe. Under the direction of various releasing hormones from the hypothalamus, the anterior pituitary makes and secretes into the bloodstream six major hormones: adrenocorticotropic hormone (ACTH), follicle-stimulating hormone (FSH), growth hormone (GH), luteinizing hormone (LH), prolactin, and thyroid-stimulating hormone (TSH). The posterior pituitary releases antidiuretic hormone (ADH) and oxytocin, both of which are made in the hypothalamus and stored in the posterior pituitary. The endocrine system also consists of additional hormone-producing glands, some of which are controlled by the hormones of the anterior pituitary. Recently, researchers have discovered that some individual cells produce hormones in response to changing conditions in the body. The other major endocrine organs are described below.

The pineal gland is found deep in the brain. For many years, its function remained a mystery. Philosopher René Descartes (1596–1650) falsely believed that the pineal was the seat of the soul and the place where thoughts were formed. Today its function is still not completely understood, but researchers know that it produces the hormone melatonin. Melatonin is involved in controlling the sleep-wake cycle and may help to regulate the reproductive cycle in females.

The thyroid gland is a butterfly-shaped tissue located in the neck just below the Adam's apple. The hypothalamus releases thyrotropin-releasing hormone (TRH), which in turn stimulates the anterior pituitary to release TSH. TSH then causes the thyroid to produce two hormones, triiodothyronine (T3) and thyroxine (T4), usually simply referred to as thyroid hormones. Thyroid hormones play a critical role in regulating almost every body function, including normal growth and development, body temperature, energy usage, digestion, heart function, sexual function, and thought patterns.

The parathyroid glands are four identical glands each about the size of a grain of rice located in the neck behind the thyroid. They function completely independently of the thyroid and produce parathyroid hormone (PTH). The only job of the parathyroids is to keep the level of calcium in the blood stable within a very narrow range. Calcium is critical to the transmission of nerve impulses, muscle contraction, and bone development.

The pancreas is a slightly flattened gland about 6 in (15 cm) long and weighing about 3 oz (85 g). It is located behind the stomach on the upper left side of the body. About 95% of the cells in the pancreas are exocrine cells that secrete digestive chemicals into a duct that empties into the small intestine. Embedded in the exocrine tissue are clumps of endocrine cells that secrete the hormones insulin and glucagon. These regulate the level of glucose (sugar) in the blood. All cells use glucose for energy. Insulin reduces the amount of glucose in the blood by opening a channel to allow glucose to enter into cells. Excess glucose is stored in the liver and skeletal muscles. Glucagon stimulates the liver to release glucose when the level in the blood is too low to meet cellular energy demands.

The adrenal glands are small triangular glands about 1.5 in high and 3 in long (3.8 × 7.6 cm) located at the top of each kidney. These glands consist of an outer cortex and an inner medulla that produce different hormones. Once again, regulation begins in the hypothalamus, where corticotropin-releasing hormone (CRH) stimulates the anterior pituitary to release adrenocorticotropic hormone (ACTH). This, in turn, causes the adrenal cortex to release cortisol, sometimes called the stress hormone. Cortisol has multiple roles in the body, including blood pressure regulation, usage of nutrients from food, and suppression of inflammation. The cortex also produces the hormone aldosterone. Aldosterone plays a role in the amount of sodium, potassium, and water that are excreted in urine when blood is filtered through the kidneys. This affects the body's fluid balance, blood pressure, and the acidity level (pH) of blood. Dehydroepiandrosterone (DHEA), also made by the cortex, is converted in male testes into testosterone and in female ovaries into estrogen.

The adrenal medulla, the inner part of the adrenal gland, produces epinephrine (also called adrenaline) and norepinephrine (also called noradrenaline). These are known as fight or flight hormones because they prepare the body for urgent action. Epinephrine increases heart rate so that more blood goes to the muscles and the brain. It also relaxes the airways to make oxygen more available. Norepinephrine increases blood pressure by narrowing blood vessels. These hormones also temporarily decrease the body's ability to feel pain. Together epinephrine and norepinephrine produce a heart-pounding, face-flushing, sweaty response to fear. Compared to other hormones, their period of effectiveness is short.

The testes are male reproductive organs. Their main functions are to produce sperm and androgens (male hormones), primarily testosterone. Testosterone is produced under the influence of gonadotropin-releasing hormone (GnRH) from the hypothalamus. This hormone then stimulates the anterior pituitary to produce FSH and LH. In men, these hormones act on the testes to stimulate them to secrete testosterone and cause sperm to mature. Testosterone stimulates the development of male secondary sexual characteristics at puberty and throughout adulthood is necessary for sperm production, sex drive, and sexual performance.

The ovaries are paired female reproductive organs located in the abdomen. Their main functions are to release eggs for fertilization and to produce estrogens (female hormones) and some progesterone. Estrogens are triggered by the same pathway as androgens in males. In females, the exact same controlling hormones—FSH and LH—that act on the testes in men, act on the ovaries in women to regulate the menstrual cycle. In the ovary, an egg matures in a sac of cells called a follicle. FSH stimulates the follicle to produce estrogens and the egg to mature. LH causes the midcycle release of a mature egg from an ovarian follicle so that it can be fertilized if sperm are present.

3. How were hormones discovered?

The concept of hormones—signaling molecules that travel through the bloodstream in tiny quantities and change the activity of tissues distant from their source—is a relatively new view of how messages move through the body. Before researchers found evidence of hormones, they believed that all signaling information moved along nerves.

The first known intentional hormone experiment was performed in 1848 using six roosters. Arnold Berthold (1803–1861), a doctor in Göttingen, Germany, removed both testicles from two roosters and one testicle from two roosters. With another two roosters, he removed both testicles, discarded one and switched the other so that neither bird got its own organ. He implanted the switched testicle in each bird's belly to see what would happen when it was not connected to its normal nerves.

The two roosters with no testicles became fat, lazy, and lost interest in chasing hens. The two roosters with one testicle acted like normal intact roosters. But to Berthold's surprise, so did the two birds with the switched testicles implanted in their bellies. When he killed the birds with the transplanted testicle, he discovered that the misplaced organ had no nerve connections but was surrounded by blood vessels. This strongly suggested that whatever messaging chemical the testicles produced, it traveled through the blood and not along nerves. Berthold published his results, but they were ignored and he did not continue his experiments.

Doctors became familiar with the symptoms of certain disorders long before they realized the causes were hormonal excesses or deficiencies. Nevertheless, some tried injecting extracts from various glands to see what changes they caused. Charles-Édouard Brown-Séquard (1817–1894) injected himself with an extract from monkey testes and claimed that it rejuvenated his sexual prowess. Despite the fact that the testes do not store testosterone and it would take hundreds of pounds of monkey testes to extract enough testosterone to have any effect, thousands of men tried this "therapy."

In the early 1900s, English physiologists Ernest Starling (1866–1927) and William Bayliss (1860–1924) set out to prove a theory by Ivan Pavlov (1849–1936) that when food entered the intestine, nerves sent a signal to the brain, causing the brain to return a signal to the pancreas to release digestive juices. After a series of rather gruesome experiments that involved cutting away the nerves around the pancreas of a dog and then stimulating its intestine with a sand and acid mixture to mimic partially digested food, Starling and Bayliss proved that Pavlov was wrong. The pancreas produced digestive juices even when all the nerves to it had been removed.

Starling and Bayliss theorized that cells in the intestine secreted a chemical messenger that traveled to the pancreas independent of nerves. This messenger then stimulated the production of digestive juices. They named the messenger "secretin" and, in 1905, came up with the word "hormone" from the Greek word *ormao*, which means "to excite" or "stir up," to describe this type of messenger.

During the next 20 years, several other hormones were identified, but the first truly dramatic breakthrough came with the isolation of insulin in 1921. Insulin must be present for the body to use glucose for energy. Before 1921 type 1 diabetes, an autoimmune disorder in which the body kills its own insulin-producing cells, was a death sentence (see question 35).

The pancreas is mainly an exocrine gland that makes digestive juice that travels through a duct and drains into the small intestine, but embedded in the exocrine gland are clumps of endocrine cells that secrete insulin into the bloodstream. In 1920, Frederick Banting (1891–1941), a poor and struggling Canadian physician, had the idea that if the exocrine cells of the pancreas were destroyed, the secretion from the endocrine cells could be isolated.

Banting was a surgeon, not a researcher, and he had no background in endocrinology. Despite this, he convinced John James Rickard Macleod (1876–1935), a scientist at the University of Toronto, to give him lab space and some dogs to experiment on. Initially, Banting and his assistant, Charles Best (1889–1978), were unsuccessful. Banting, however, remained obsessed with his idea and persisted despite many setbacks. Eventually, when some of his results looked promising, a biochemist, James Collip (1892–1965), joined the team to help isolate the endocrine substance.

The men working to isolate insulin were not a happy team. From the start, Macleod and Banting disliked each other. Banting, a farm boy, thought that upper class Macleod looked down on him and accused Macleod of taking credit for his and Best's research. In addition, just when success appeared possible, Banting and Collip became so estranged that they could not be left alone in the same room. They physically fought and had to be separated by Best on at least two occasions. Nevertheless, on January 11, 1922, 14-year-old diabetic Leonard Thompson, who was just days away from dying, received an injection of insulin extract. The injection worked. With regular insulin shots, Thompson lived another 13 years and died of pneumonia.

Success did not improve the relationship among the team members. When Banting and Macleod were awarded the Nobel Prize in 1923, neither attended the ceremony because they did not want to stand on the stage with each other. Since 1922, insulin has sustained the lives of millions of diabetics. Initially, it was extracted from pork and beef pancreases. Since 1983, it has been made in the laboratory using genetically engineered *E. coli* bacteria or yeast cells.

With the success of insulin, interest in hormones soared. Harvey Cushing (1869–1939), a Yale brain surgeon, made the connection between a secretion from the pituitary (adrenocorticotropic hormone) and the regulation of cortisol produced by the adrenal cortex. In 1927, the chemical structure of thyroid hormone was determined, and in 1931, thyroid-stimulating hormone was isolated from cow thyroids. Edward Doisy (1893–1986) isolated estrogen in 1929. Testosterone was isolated in 1935 and quickly synthesized in the laboratory, a contribution that won the synthesizers the 1939 Nobel Prize in Chemistry.

Despite all these advances, hormones are effective in only such tiny quantities that no tests sensitive enough to measure their concentration in the blood existed until 1959 when Rosalyn Yalow, a nuclear physicist, along with two colleagues, developed a testing technique called radioimmunoassay. This breakthrough allowed endocrinologists to measure quantities as small as one-trillionth of a gram of hormone in one milliliter of blood. Radioimmunoassay, still widely used today, won Yalow the Nobel

Prize in 1977. She was only the second woman to win in physiology or medicine. Many life-changing developments have resulted from the ability to accurately measure hormones. One was development of oral contraceptives in 1960, and a second was the success of in vitro fertilization in 1978.

Researchers continue to find new hormones as well as explore the mechanisms by which they activate changes in cells. Aaron Lerner (1920–2007), a Yale University dermatologist, discovered melatonin in 1958, although the hormone was not seriously researched until the 1980s. Jeffrey Friedman (1954–) discovered leptin, a weight-control hormone, in 1994. To his surprise, he found that it is synthesized in individual fat cells. Ghrelin, which stimulates both appetite and the release of growth hormone from the pituitary, was identified in 1999.

More recently, a hormone called asprosin was discovered in 2016 by researchers at Baylor College of Medicine. This hormone is involved in the release of glucose from the liver. It is found in unusually high levels in people with type 2 diabetes, a fact that researchers hope may lead to new treatments for the disorder. As of 2022, more than 50 hormones and signaling molecules have been identified. Many are produced by individual cells rather than endocrine organs, and their functions remain incompletely understood.

4. How does my body know when to secrete hormones?

A major role of hormones is to maintain homeostasis in the body. The word "homeostasis" is derived from two ancient Greek words, *homeo* meaning "similar to" and *stasis* meaning "standing still." In other words, homeostasis is the condition of maintaining a set point or equilibrium for internal body functions. To do this, sensors throughout the body constantly monitor internal functions such as temperature, blood pressure, and blood concentration of glucose, sodium, potassium, and calcium, all of which must remain within a very narrow range for the body to stay healthy.

Most hormones maintain homeostasis through negative feedback loops. In a negative feedback loop, the response to an initial stimulus is reduced. For example, in a healthy person, the concentration of glucose in the blood is kept within a narrow range. When food is digested, glucose is absorbed into the bloodstream. Rising levels of glucose (high blood sugar, the initial stimulus) signal endocrine cells in the pancreas called beta cells to secrete the hormone insulin. Insulin opens a channel into cells so that glucose can leave the blood and be used for cellular energy. It also allows excess glucose to be stored in the liver.

As glucose enters cells or is stored, its concentration in the blood drops (the stimulus of high blood sugar is reduced). When the amount of glucose falls below a certain set point, insulin secretion stops. When blood glucose levels drop below the set point (low blood sugar, a new initial stimulus), another group of endocrine cells in the pancreas called alpha cells begins to secrete the hormone glucagon. Glucagon travels through the bloodstream and signals the liver to release stored glucose in order to increase the amount of glucose in the blood and return it to the set point (the stimulus of low blood sugar is reduced). When enough glucose has been released by the liver or the person eats again, glucagon production stops, and insulin production starts. See question 34 to find out what happens when this feedback cycle fails.

Many sensors in the body send their information to the hypothalamus, an organ in the brain that links the nervous and endocrine systems. For example, when a person exercises heavily, the body loses water. This causes the concentration of sodium ions in the blood that are critical for maintaining fluid balance to increase. The increase is registered by specialized nerve cells in the hypothalamus that signal the posterior pituitary to release antidiuretic hormone (ADH) and to activate thirst sensors. ADH acts on the kidneys, triggering them to conserve water and excrete more sodium so that the blood returns to its set point. The result is the production of a small quantity of concentrated urine. On the other hand, if a person drinks a large amount of liquid, secretion of ADH stops, and the kidneys return the body to equilibrium by producing a large amount of dilute urine. To learn how drinking alcohol upsets this balance, see question 40.

Most hormones are part of negative feedback cycles, but prolactin production is an example of a positive feedback cycle. In a positive feedback cycle, response to the initial stimulus is intensified. Prolactin is a hormone that causes a woman to make breast milk. When a baby nurses (the initial stimulus), nerves activated by the baby's sucking send a message to the hypothalamus that causes the anterior pituitary to release more prolactin. The more the baby sucks, the more prolactin is released, and the more milk the mother makes (the response to the stimulus is intensified). When a baby stops nursing, no prolactin is produced, and the mother's milk supply dries up.

Not all hormonal secretion is stimulated by internal conditions. External factors can stimulate the secretion of epinephrine, norepinephrine, and melatonin. Epinephrine and norepinephrine are released rapidly when a person feels threatened and may need to respond to an external situation by either fighting or running away. The release of melatonin, a hormone associated with sleep cycles, is connected to the amount of light entering the eye. As the environment becomes darker and less light enters the eye, signals are sent by the optic nerve that result in the production of more melatonin. To learn how this affects teenagers' sleep patterns, see question 32.

5. How do hormones know which cells to target?

Hormones are powerful chemicals that moderate all types of vital activities, from maintaining body temperature to signaling hunger to stimulating sexual behavior. They are effective in tiny quantities of parts per billion. Although their job is to keep the body in equilibrium, researchers have recently discovered that many hormones are secreted in short bursts rather than continuously.

Once released into the bloodstream, a hormone comes in contact with almost every cell in the body. The hormone does not seek out particular cells, but instead tends to "bump into" cells that respond to it. A few hormones such as thyroid hormone, which mediates metabolism, or insulin, which allows glucose to enter cells to be used for energy, affect all cells. Nevertheless, many hormones can cause different changes in different types of cells (see question 6) or affect the same cells differently at different stages in the life cycle. Any cell that a hormone acts on is called a target cell. Target cells have receptors that allow them to interact with specific hormones and ignore other hormones in the bloodstream.

Hormones can be classified as either lipophilic (fat loving) or hydrophilic (water loving). This difference is important because it affects the way in which a hormone activates changes in the target cell. Lipophilic hormones, which include sex hormones and thyroid hormones, cannot dissolve in blood, which is mostly water. To be carried through the bloodstream to reach their target cells, lipophilic hormones must bond to a water-loving protein that "hides" part of the hormone molecule and allows it to be carried by blood.

When a lipophilic hormone meets a target cell receptor, it uncouples from the water-loving protein. Cell membranes contain fat. Once the fat-loving hormone has ditched the water-loving protein that allowed it to use the blood for transportation, it dissolves into the fat of the cell membrane and crosses into the cell's cytoplasm. A receptor in the cytoplasm then binds with the hormone, and this receptor-hormone complex acts on the cell nucleus to change the cell's activity. Because the hormone itself enters the cell, the hormone is called the primary messenger.

Hydrophilic (or water loving), hormones such as insulin, are made of chains of amino acids. These hormones can dissolve in water. Since blood is about 50% water, hydrophilic hormones have no trouble moving through the circulatory system until they encounter their target cells.

Once a water-loving hormone recognizes a target cell, it cannot simply dissolve through the fatty cell membrane. Instead, it binds to a receptor on the target cell's surface. The act of binding changes the receptor's shape. This shape change triggers a series of chemical reactions in the membrane that produce what is called a secondary messenger. The hormone itself never enters the cell. Instead, the secondary messenger enters the cytoplasm, undergoes a number of chemical reactions, and ultimately changes the cell's activity such as causing it to make a new protein or to stop making a protein. Certain chemicals can block receptors and/or interfere with the production of secondary messengers and enzymes needed for the cell to "read" the hormonal message. These chemicals are called endocrine disruptors, and they are discussed in question 38.

6. Do men and women make the same hormones?

For many years, testosterone was considered an exclusively male hormone. Estrogens (there are several kinds, the most prominent being estradiol) were considered exclusively female. We now know, however, that for good health, both men and women need a balance of both estrogen and testosterone. At puberty, these sex hormones help the reproductive organs mature. In adults, they are essential for sexual performance and reproduction.

Sex hormones are made in the reproductive organs in both men and women. In addition, the adrenal cortex makes testosterone, estrogen, and progesterone in both sexes, but the amounts are miniscule compared to the quantity produced by reproductive organs. Whether they are made in men or women, testosterone is masculinizing, and estrogen is feminizing. The different physical effects they produce are caused by the quantity of each hormone made and the cells each acts on.

Men make about 20 times more testosterone than women, 95% of which is made in the testes. The process starts when the hypothalamus releases gonadotropin-releasing hormone (GnRH). GnRH signals the anterior pituitary gland to release follicle-stimulating hormone (FSH) and luteinizing hormone (LH). In adult men, LH stimulates cells in the testes to produce testosterone. FSH aids in the production of sperm.

Men do not directly synthesize estrogen. Instead, they form it through the breakdown of testosterone. This conversion is achieved by an enzyme called aromatase that is found in cells in men's adrenal glands, testes, adipose (fat) tissue, and brain. A balance between estrogen and testosterone is necessary to maintain sex drive, erectile function, a proper balance between muscle and fat, and development and maintenance of strong bones. Both too much and too little estrogen can cause loss of male sex drive, erectile dysfunction, fatigue, mood swings, anxiety, and depression. Too much estrogen can also cause development of male breasts (gynecomastia), and too little can cause bone loss and weight gain.

In women, the same hypothalamus and pituitary hormones are released, but FSH regulates the maturation of an egg in the ovary and stimulates estrogen production. LH stimulates the ovary to produce an estrogen burst that causes the midcycle release of a mature egg from an ovarian follicle. After the egg has been released, the remains of the follicle (now called the corpus luteum) produce progesterone to thicken the uterus lining to prepare for implantation of a fertilized egg.

The ovaries also produce a small amount of testosterone, but almost all of it is converted into estrogen. Exercise can increase a woman's testosterone production. This can be a problem for any female athlete who already has a higher-than-average production of testosterone. Testosterone supplements, along with other anabolic steroids, are banned performance-enhancing drugs and are tested for in elite athletic competitions. One example of what can happen when a woman athlete has a naturally high amount of testosterone is discussed in case illustration 5.

Too much testosterone in women is one symptom of polycystic ovary syndrome (PCOS). In PCOS, the ovary is filled with small cysts, and fertility is often impaired. Women may develop facial hair, acne, and a tendency to become obese. They also are likely to develop insulin resistance, which leads to type 2 diabetes (see question 35). Some other early research suggests that excess androgens in men may also cause increased insulin resistance.

Three other hormones have traditionally been considered female hormones. Oxytocin, which in women stimulates contractions when giving birth and promotes bonding with the baby, is also found in men and may encourage social bonding. Men also make small amounts of prolactin, the hormone that stimulates milk production in new mothers, but its function in men is not clear. Relaxin, a hormone that relaxes muscles and joints in women in preparation for giving birth, is also made in men and may be involved in sperm motility. Even the hormone human chorionic gonadotropin (hCG), which is associated with the production of progesterone in pregnant women, is made in small quantities by men and nonpregnant women. Although men and women make the same hormones, they make then in different quantities, and these hormones often act on different tissues in men and women or act at different times.

Growth and Development

7. What is growth hormone, and what role does it play in the body?

Growth hormone (GH), also called somatotropin, is a hormone produced by the pituitary that modifies metabolism. Along with other hormones, it helps keep the body in a stable state by adjusting energy use by cells. Growth is a complex process, and GH is part of an extensive web of hormones and hormonelike chemicals that act on every tissue in the body to regulate energy balance and growth. Researchers are still unraveling the multiple roles of GH in the body.

In the late 1800s, doctors figured out that a functioning pituitary was necessary for children to reach a normal height, but GH itself was not isolated until 1956, and its chemical structure was not deciphered until 1972. Initially, GH to treat GH-deficient children had to be extracted from pituitaries collected from human cadavers. This meant the supply of GH was extremely limited, so in the early 1960s, the National Pituitary Agency was formed to supervise GH treatment in the United States. Between 1963 and 1985, about 7,700 American children were treated for severe short stature due to GH deficiency.

Disaster struck the GH program in 1985. Ten or more years after some of the children had been treated with cadaver-derived GH, they developed Creutzfeldt-Jakob disease (CJD), sometimes called mad cow disease. CJD is a rare, always fatal, brain disease that rapidly progresses to loss of mental and physical functions followed by death. The cause is a prion, which is an infectious protein. In these children, the prion had been transmitted by GH extract from some infected cadavers. Cadaver pituitaries could no longer be used.

Fortunately, Genentech, a biotechnology company specializing in recombinant DNA technology, had in 1981 cloned the gene that regulates production of GH in the pituitary. This allowed them to develop safe laboratory-produced GH. Manufactured GH became available in large quantities, resulting in the development of many nonmedical products containing the hormone. These products are advertised as having anti-aging and performance-enhancing properties, although they have repeatedly been shown to be of little or no value. The U.S. Food and Drug Administration (FDA) has not approved any human nonprescription uses of GH. When used by athletes with or without a prescription to boost muscle mass, GH is illegal (see question 8).

The only other GH product approved by the FDA is a form of GH specifically for cattle. It is used to increase milk production. This hormone is called bovine growth hormone (BGH), or alternately, bovine somatotropin (BST). Its use is controversial. Some milk is specifically labeled as BHG- or BST-free for consumers who prefer milk from untreated cows.

Just as growth is a complicated process, the actions of GH are complicated. GH is made in the anterior pituitary, but its release into the bloodstream is controlled by the hypothalamus, a pea-sized bit of neural tissue in the brain. The hypothalamus makes growth hormone-releasing hormone (GHRH) that stimulates the anterior pituitary to make and secrete GH. GH is not released continuously. It enters the bloodstream in spurts every three to five hours, with about 75% of each day's production released during sleep.

The amount of GH secreted by the anterior pituitary varies throughout the life cycle. The hormone appears to have little effect on fetal development, although researchers do not know why. Especially large amounts are released around puberty when the body undergoes major growth and shape changes. The amount of GH naturally decreases as a person ages; however, adults continue to need GH in small amounts. The role of GH in adults is not well understood, but it is thought to affect cholesterol levels, bone density, heart health, and psychological well-being.

The most obvious physical effect of GH is to increase the height of children and height and muscle mass in adolescents. This occurs in part because GH is anabolic, meaning it stimulates increased protein synthesis. In addition to height and muscle, GH stimulates the growth of internal organs, including the brain. GH also helps strengthen bones by increasing the amount of calcium retained by the body and incorporated into bone. It further modifies metabolism by helping to maintain fluid balance and blood glucose levels.

Although GH acts on many tissues, most of its effects occur indirectly rather than through direct interaction between cells and the hormone. An exception is the effect GH has on fat cells where direct interaction between the fat cell and GH prevents fat cells from taking in lipids (fats) circulating in the blood. GH also stimulates the liver and some other tissues directly, causing them to produce a hormonelike chemical called insulin-like growth factor 1 (IGF-1). The interaction between IGF-1 and many tissues causes cells to increase in both size and number, an example of the indirect effect of GH. IGF-I is also part of a complex system that maintains homeostasis, including affecting the glucose level in the blood and fluid balance.

Like most hormones, GH secretion is controlled by a negative feedback loop. The hypothalamus receives information from sensors in the body that detect changes such as the level of IGF-1, blood glucose, and the amount of circulating GH. When hormone levels become too high, the hypothalamus makes growth hormone-inhibiting hormone (GHIH), also called somatostatin (not to be confused with somatotropin, the alternate name for GH). When GHIH is released from the hypothalamus, it prevents the release of GH from the anterior pituitary. Together, these two hormones made by the hypothalamus act in opposition to each other to form a negative feedback loop that controls growth and helps maintain blood homeostasis (for more on feedback loops, see question 4).

8. What happens when you have too much or too little growth hormone?

Growth hormone (GH), produced in the anterior pituitary under stimulation of growth hormone-releasing hormone (GHRH) made by the hypothalamus, helps maintain chemical balance in the body. Because GH directly or indirectly affects every tissue, any deviation from normal levels causes serious physical and biochemical changes in the body. The types of changes depend on the age at which the deficiency or excess occurs.

GH deficiency in children causes what is medically called proportionate dwarfism, although the preferred social term is short stature. A person with proportionate short stature has a height of 4 ft 10 in (147 cm) or less when growth is complete, with a trunk and limbs that are in the correct size relationship. The most common cause of proportionate dwarfism is a defect in the GH system. Disproportionate dwarfism, in which the trunk and limbs are mismatched in size, is caused by various genetic defects unrelated to GH deficiency.

Deficits in the GH can occur at any of several levels. The hypothalamus may fail to produce adequate GHRH. The pituitary may fail to respond to GHRH. The pituitary may release adequate GH, but the liver may fail to produce adequate insulin-like growth factor 1 (IGF-1). IGF-1 is responsible for many of the indirect effects of GH. Finally, tissues may not adequately respond to IGF-1, and as a result, they fail to grow. Very rarely, a tumor in the hypothalamus will produce excess growth hormone-inhibiting hormone (GHIH). This hormone blocks the pituitary from producing GH. In any of these situations, the result is short stature.

GH deficit in children can be treated most successfully when diagnosed early. Warning signs that could trigger testing include height below the third percentile on the childhood growth chart, slower than normal growth, and in older children, very delayed puberty, or no sexual development at all. After an abundance of tests to check each step in GH regulation, an endocrinologist may prescribe injections of GH. Daily injections are given below the skin but above the muscle (subcutaneously), usually in the abdomen. GH cannot be taken as a pill because it is inactivated in the stomach. Because many people consider being tall a cultural advantage, some parents of short but normal, healthy children pressure doctors to prescribe growth hormone. The use of GH that is not medically necessary is illegal and a prescribing physician's license to practice medicine could be suspended.

The degree to which supplemental GH increases height and organ development depends on how soon treatment is begun. Treatment continues until the long bones in the body stop growing, usually around age 18 in women and 21 in men. Relatively new research suggests that people with childhood GH deficiency benefit from some continued GH treatment as adults.

There is a natural decline of 1%–2% a year in GH production in adults. For quite a while, endocrinologists thought that since adults were no longer growing taller, GH was not needed. Research now suggests that adults need to produce some GH and can become GH deficient. Much less is known about GH deficiency in adults than in children, but research suggests that adults who are GH deficient have lower levels of HDL or "good" cholesterol, are inclined to gain weight, have high blood glucose levels, tend to develop type 2 diabetes, have other metabolic imbalances, often are low energy, and experience a high level of anxiety and depression.

Since it is unclear what a "normal" level of GH is at various adult ages, treatment of adults with GH remains controversial with one exception. GH is approved to treat muscle wasting in adults with HIV/AIDS. The HIV virus has been shown to directly disrupt GH function, leading to loss of muscle.

Excess GH production is extremely rare in children. When it occurs, the condition is called gigantism, and children grow to a great height. The tallest person on record is Robert Wadlow (1918–1940), an Illinois man who grew to be 8 ft 11 in (272 cm), weighed 490 lb (223 kg), and wore a size 37 shoe. Wadlow was normal-sized at birth but soon began to grow rapidly. He died at age 22, not from a condition related to his size, but from an infection. Only about 100 cases of gigantism have been documented. It is thought the condition is due to mutated genes that allow the overproduction of IGF-1.

Excess GH in adults produces a disorder called acromegaly. Because adult bones cannot elongate, people with this condition develop swollen hands and feet. Their lips, nose, and tongue enlarge. The brow becomes more prominent. Their jaw juts forward, and the space between the teeth increases. People with acromegaly also develop thick, coarse, oily skin and sweat excessively. They may feel weak and easily fatigued. Tests often show high levels of blood glucose and other metabolic abnormalities.

Acromegaly develops gradually over years and is not often diagnosed before middle age. The disorder is rare. Only three or four new cases per one million population occur each year. They are usually caused by a benign (noncancerous) pituitary tumor. Some tumors can be surgically removed. Drugs that block the action of the hormone secreted by the tumor may be used when surgery is not possible. Death in people with acromegaly usually is caused by cardiovascular or metabolic abnormalities resulting from excess GH.

Another way in which people can be exposed to excess GH is by using GH injections when they are not GH deficient. This is an illegal use. The main consumers of illegal GH are athletes, bodybuilders, and aging adults. In the United States, GH is regulated under the 1990 Anabolic Steroids Control Act (see question 39 for more on anabolic steroids). The Act states that distribution and possession with intent to distribute "for any . . . use other than the treatment of a disease or other recognized medical condition" is a felony with up to five years of prison time (Drug Enforcement Administration 2019). GH is recognized as a prohibited performance-enhancing drug by the World Anti-Doping Agency, United States Anti-Doping Agency, International Olympic Committee, and many professional sports leagues. The National Basketball Association and Major League Baseball both measure GH in their blood tests for banned performance-enhancing drugs.

Studies of the potential benefit of GH to adults who are not hormone deficient are contradictory and often fail to meet the standards of professional medical research. The attraction is that some studies found that GH injections increased lean muscle mass and decreased body fat by about 4.4 lb (2 kg); however, athletic performance did not improve. In addition, increased muscle mass comes at a high price. Common side effects include fluid retention, joint and muscle pain, development of breasts in men, increased risk of developing type 2 diabetes, and increased risk of certain cancers. And GH is expensive, costing anywhere between $800 and $5,000 per month.

To get around the issue of legality, many products are advertised as containing "GH releasers" that stimulate the body to make more GH or that theoretically are transformed by the body into GH. For example, as this book was being written, a television commercial was airing for an antiaging face cream that claimed to contain "GH releasers" that would make a person look and feel younger. In reality, the only way to get GH into the body is by daily injection. Any GH or so-called releasers taken by mouth are inactivated in the stomach, nor can GH or "releasers" in gels, sprays, creams, or patches cross through the skin and into the body.

Legal use of GH requires both a doctor's prescription and supervision, with the need for GH backed up by laboratory testing. GH bought over the Internet is illegal, even when a doctor has written prescription for it, because the law requires a physician to directly supervise its use in an ongoing fashion. In addition, black market GH, from Internet sources, may contain contaminants—or no GH at all.

9. Why will drinking milk give you strong bones?

Milk is a wonder fluid when it comes to making strong bones. One 8 oz cup (237 mL) of cow's milk contains 300 mg of calcium, an essential element for building strong bones, transmitting nerve impulses, allowing muscles to contract, and helping blood to clot. Cheese, yogurt, and other dairy products are also good sources of calcium, but plant milk such as almond, soy, and rice milk are not unless they have been fortified with added calcium by the manufacturer. Some breakfast cereals and fruit juices also contain added calcium. The amount of calcium a person needs depends on age. People aged 9–18 years need 1,300 mg daily, the highest amount of any age group.

Bone is living material that acts as a calcium bank for the body. About 99% of calcium is found in bones and teeth in the form of an insoluble complex of calcium and phosphate called hydroxyapatite. The remaining 1% circulates in the blood as the positively charged ion Ca^+. Under the control of several hormones, small amounts of bone are constantly built up or broken down to keep the calcium level stable within an extremely narrow range.

The process of building up and breaking down bone is called bone remodeling. During childhood, more calcium is deposited in bones and more hydroxyapatite is formed than is destroyed, so bones grow both larger and stronger. As a person matures, the rate of calcium deposit gradually declines. After a relatively stable period in midlife when bone formation and destruction are about equal, bone destruction increases, resulting in about a 1% loss of bone mass each year. As a result, bones in the elderly are less dense and more easily broken, a condition called osteoporosis.

Parathyroid hormone (PTH) is the most important hormone controlling the blood concentration of calcium. PTH is produced by the parathyroid glands. These are rice-sized, mustard-yellow glands located in the neck, behind, but independent of, the thyroid gland. Most people have four parathyroid glands, but individuals can be healthy with as many as six or as few as one. These glands were first described in a rhinoceros in 1852, but it took a century to locate them in humans, and a complete description was not made until 1980.

Blood passes continuously through the parathyroid glands, which contain sensors whose only job is to monitor the concentration of calcium ions. These sensors allow the parathyroids to rapidly adjust the amount of PTH secreted into the bloodstream. When the sensors register a drop in circulating calcium, the glands release PTH. This starts the process of bone destruction and the release of calcium ions into the blood.

Bone remodeling is a complex, multistep process. The short version is that PTH activates a type of bone cell called an osteoclast. Osteoclasts are able to tunnel into bone and secrete acid and enzymes that break down hydroxyapatite, the mineralized (hard) part of bone. This ultimately results in the release calcium ions and phosphate ions.

Normally (for abnormal situations, see question 11), only a tiny amount of hydroxyapatite is dissolved. It is enough to bring calcium levels back to their set point but not enough to weaken the bone. At the same time, PTH acts on the kidney so that more calcium is retained, and more phosphate is excreted in urine. Vitamin D also plays a role in increasing the amount of calcium absorbed from the small intestine (see question 10).

A second hormone called calcitonin acts in opposition to PTH, although its effects are much weaker than PTH. Calcitonin was discovered in 1962 by Canadian biochemist Douglas Copp (1915–1998). Copp originally thought that calcitonin was produced by the parathyroids, but later it was discovered that this hormone is made by specialized C-cells embedded in the thyroid gland. Calcitonin is found in animals, from fish to mammals, and appears to reduce calcium levels in the body. The way it works is still not completely understood. It appears to activate bone cells called osteoblasts. These cells come together and as a group lay down collagen, a flexible protein matrix, on the surface of the bone. They then produce substances that cause calcium to be deposited into the collagen to mineralize it and make new bone. Calcitonin also increases excretion of calcium by the kidney.

10. What does vitamin D have to do with calcium and bone growth?

Vitamins are compounds that are not made by the body but that in tiny quantities are essential for normal growth, development, and cell functioning. To remain healthy, vitamins must be acquired from diet. For years, scientists considered vitamin D only a vitamin. Today, it is recognized as both a vitamin and a hormone that is involved in calcium regulation, bone development, and bone maintenance.

Rickets is a disorder that causes soft bones and poor skeletal development in children. The adult version is called osteomalacia, or literally, "bone sickness." The disorder was recognized in the 1600s, although its cause was unknown. By the early 1900s, people had figured out that eating citrus fruits prevented scurvy (a vitamin C deficiency) and brown rice prevented beriberi (a B1 deficiency). These findings motivated scientists to search for a food that would prevent rickets. By the 1920s they had found that food—a daily teaspoon of cod liver oil. Later rickets was identified as being caused by vitamin D deficiency. At about the same time, other researchers discovered that exposure to sunlight would also prevent rickets because small amounts can be synthesized when ultraviolet radiation penetrates the skin. Vitamin D was isolated in the 1930s and soon began to be produced synthetically, but it remained unclear whether vitamin D was a true vitamin that had to be acquired from an outside source or a hormone that the body could make.

Vitamin D, whose chemical structure is related to the cholesterol molecule, comes in several forms. Vitamin D$_2$ is the form absorbed from natural food sources. It is present in only a few foods, mainly fatty fish such as tuna, cod, and salmon. Because less than 10% of a person's vitamin D requirement comes from natural food sources, countries as diverse as the United States, Canada, India, and Finland have required that common foods, including most cow's milk, soy and other plant milks, breakfast cereals, some orange juice, yogurt, and margarine, be fortified with added vitamin D. Human breast milk is so deficient in vitamin D that exclusively breastfed babies should be given daily vitamin D supplements for normal bone development.

Vitamin D$_3$ is made when ultraviolet B sunlight (UVB) strikes bare skin. Most people do not make enough vitamin D from sun exposure to meet their body's needs. Clothing blocks UVB light, as does the use of sunscreen. UVB is also blocked by window glass. Dark skin absorbs less UVB than light skin.

In the United States, the daily recommended dietary allowance (RDA) of vitamin D for people aged 1–70 is 15 micrograms (mcg) or its equivalent, 600 international units (IUs). Some professional organizations recommend higher amounts, but many people fail to meet even the lower RDA level. Nevertheless, most physicians agree that protecting against excessive sun exposure to avoid an increased risk of skin cancer is more important than increasing the skin's production of vitamin D, especially because vitamin is added to many common foods.

Both vitamin D from diet and vitamin D made by skin are inactive until they go through two chemical transformations, first in the liver and then in the kidney. The active form of vitamin D is called calcitriol, and it is considered a hormone. Most calcium is absorbed in the duodenum, the part of the small intestine closest to the stomach. However, calcium cannot leave the duodenum by itself. It needs to bind with a carrier protein called calbindin to transport it across the duodenum wall and into the bloodstream. This is where vitamin D comes into the picture. In its active form, it switches on the gene that makes the carrier protein. As the amount of carrier protein increases, the amount of calcium moved from the duodenum into the bloodstream increases, and thus vitamin D helps to increase calcium absorption. This ability to move calcium is why calcium and vitamin D are often combined in dietary supplements. Vitamin D also activates bone cells, and, in actions unrelated to bones, it plays a role in developing immunity and regulating cell division.

II. What happens if you have too much or too little of the hormones regulating calcium and bone growth?

A healthy 154 lb (70 kg) person has about 2.6 lb (1.2 kg) of calcium in their body, 99% of which is stored in the bones and teeth. The remainder circulates in the blood as positively charged ions. Circulating calcium plays an essential role in nerve conduction, muscle contraction, blood clotting, fluid regulation, and the maintenance of strong, dense bones.

The primary role of parathyroid hormone (PTH) is to keep the concentration of circulating calcium within a very narrow range. PTH is aided in this by the hormone vitamin D and, to a lesser degree, the hormone calcitonin. These hormones act on the kidneys to regulate the amount of calcium excreted in urine, on the digestive system to control the amount of calcium absorbed from digested food, and on bones to manage the depositing or withdrawal of calcium. When things go wrong, hypercalcemia or hypocalcemia can occur.

Hypercalcemia is the condition of having too high a concentration of calcium in the blood. People have four tiny parathyroid glands located behind the thyroid gland in the neck. These glands produce PTH, the primary hormone regulating calcium concentration. More than 90% of cases of hypercalcemia are caused by tumors of the parathyroid glands that cause them to overproduce PTH. Often these tumors are benign (noncancerous). Surgery to remove the overactive gland cures 95% of these cases.

Other causes of hypercalcemia include cancers that invade the bone and cause the release of calcium, advanced kidney disease, and taking large amounts vitamin D as a supplement. Vitamin D raises the level of calcium in the body by increasing its absorption from the digestive tract (see question 10). Hypercalcemia can also be caused by taking certain medications and by a few rare inherited diseases.

Symptoms of hypercalcemia may be mild and general. They often go unnoticed or are attributed to other causes, but the disorder is estimated to occur in 1 or 2 of every 1,000 adults in the United States. Symptoms include muscle weakness and joint pain, increased thirst and urination, fatigue, depression, loss of appetite, and nausea. Serious symptoms include confusion, dehydration, kidney stones, heart rhythm irregularities, and coma. When symptoms are mild, hypercalcemia is often diagnosed incidentally when blood tests are done for other reasons.

Hypocalcemia is the condition of having too little calcium in the blood. The top causes in order are long-term (chronic) or short-term (acute) kidney failure, vitamin D deficiency, magnesium deficiency, and inadequate production of PTH by the parathyroid glands. Hypocalcemia can also be caused by some hereditary disorders and may be a side effect of a chronic gastrointestinal disorder such as Crohn's disease. Although the hormone calcitonin, produced by C-cells embedded in the thyroid gland, reduces calcium levels in the blood, it appears that excess calcitonin plays little or no role in causing hypocalcemia in humans.

A diet poor in calcium does not usually result in low blood levels of calcium because the body sacrifices bone calcium in order to keep the blood level of calcium constant (see question 9). When there is not enough calcium in the diet, PTH activates cells called osteoclasts that cause bone to dissolve. This releases calcium ions into the blood. Rickets is the result of a diet chronically low in calcium in children. It causes weakened, soft, bendable bones. In adults and people with anorexia nervosa, the result is osteoporosis where bones become less dense and are easily broken. Osteoporosis causes no obvious symptoms, although it can be diagnosed with a bone density scan. The elderly are particularly susceptible to bone loss, resulting in broken bones. They usually benefit from daily supplemental calcium and vitamin D.

Pregnant women also need extra calcium and vitamin D, along with other micronutrients that promote healthy development of the fetus. There is an old saying that a woman loses a tooth with every baby. Researchers today have found there is some truth to this statement, as pregnant women have more dental problems than nonpregnant women of the same age, presumably because the fetus's need for calcium to build its own bones weakens the mother's teeth. Pregnant women are encouraged to take special prenatal vitamins formulated to meet the growing fetus's needs so that a woman does not need to sacrifice her teeth or develop weakened bones to bear a healthy child.

Reproductive Hormones across the Life Span

12. What are the predominantly female reproductive hormones?

Sex hormones develop and maintain the reproductive system. They are responsible for the physical changes that occur during puberty. In addition to regulating reproduction, these hormones also affect bone density, muscle development, fat storage, blood clotting, metabolism, social behavior, and sexual desire.

Estrogen (also spelled oestrogen) is the chief female sex hormone. It is classified as a steroid sex hormone, as are progesterone and testosterone, two other sex hormones. These hormones are all derived from changes to the cholesterol molecule and can be considered structural cousins. Women naturally produce three forms of estrogen. When people refer to "estrogen," they usually do not distinguish among the different types.

Most estrogen is made and secreted by the ovaries, although some is made by the adrenal cortex and also by fat cells. The dominant and most active form of estrogen is estradiol (also spelled oestradiol or called E2). It stimulates the changes that occur in a girl's body during puberty (see question 13). After puberty, it causes the maturation and release of the egg during the menstrual cycle (see question 15). Estrogen also has non-reproductive functions such as helping regulate cholesterol levels and fat storage and maintaining strong bones and healthy skin. In 1933, estradiol was the last form of estrogen to be isolated and its chemical structure identified.

Small amounts of estriol (oestriol or E3), another type of estrogen, are produced all the time by the ovary, but the amount increases a thousand-fold during pregnancy when estriol is secreted by the placenta. Estriol helps the uterus grow, and in some way not quite clear to researchers, it promotes healthy development of the fetus. It also helps prepare a pregnant woman's body for labor and breastfeeding. The amount of estriol in a pregnant woman begins rising at eight weeks and peaks about three weeks before delivery. Measuring the amount of estriol in a pregnant woman's urine is one way doctors can evaluate the health of the developing fetus. If a woman's estriol level peaks early instead of about three weeks before delivery, it indicates she may have a preterm delivery.

In 1929, estrone (oestrone or E1) was the first type of estrogen to be isolated and purified. It is a weak hormone, about 10 times weaker than estradiol, and is considered a minor female sex steroid. In the body, estrone is transformed into estradiol. However, it remains important because it is the only form of estrogen a woman makes after menopause. Synthetic estrone is used in some medications to treat symptoms of menopause.

Progesterone is the other major female sex hormone. It prepares the uterus for implantation of a fertilized egg by increasing the number of blood vessels growing into the uterus wall. If pregnancy occurs, increased blood flow to the uterus is necessary to maintain the pregnancy and nourish the developing fetus.

During the menstrual cycle, progesterone is produced by the corpus luteum, a structure that develops from a follicle (a growth sac) that has just released an egg from the ovary. If the egg is not fertilized, the corpus luteum stops secreting progesterone, and the uterine lining is shed (menstruation). If a fertilized egg implants in the uterus, the corpus luteum keeps secreting progesterone to support the pregnancy until the placenta develops enough to take over making the hormone. A high level of progesterone maintains the pregnancy, but it also prevents the ovary from releasing any more eggs so that fertilization of additional eggs will not happen while a woman is pregnant. Small amounts of progesterone are also produced by the adrenal cortex independent of pregnancy.

Some female hormones are produced primarily in connection with pregnancy. These hormones are protein hormones, not sex steroids, and they are essential to pregnancy. The first to be produced is human chorionic gonadotropin (hCG). Production of this hormone begins at fertilization and allows the corpus luteum to keep secreting progesterone until the placenta develops. The presence of hCG in a woman's urine is one way to determine if she is pregnant (see question 19 for more on pregnancy tests). Although hCG is primarily a hormone of pregnancy, both men and non-pregnant women make low levels of the hormone throughout their lives.

Relaxin is a hormone secreted at first by the corpus luteum and the ovary and later in pregnancy by the placenta. Initially it prevents contractions in the uterus so that implantation of a fertilized egg can take place. Toward the end of pregnancy, it softens the cervix and relaxes ligaments attached to the pelvis to make delivery easier.

Oxytocin is a hormone associated with labor and delivery. It is secreted by the posterior pituitary. During labor, it stimulates uterine contractions. It also plays a role in bonding between the mother and newborn. Small amounts of this hormone are also made by men in whom it also is thought to promote social bonding.

Prolactin, a hormone secreted by the anterior pituitary, causes breasts to increase in size during pregnancy and prepares them to produce milk. The action of a baby nursing stimulates more prolactin secretion in order to maintain the mother's milk supply.

13. What physical changes occur during puberty in girls?

During puberty, a girl's body changes into a woman's body. This period stretches over about four years and for most girls begins between ages 9 and 13. Puberty is a time of great physical, emotional, social, and hormonal change. By the end of puberty, a girl has become a woman who can become pregnant and have a baby.

The physical changes in a girl's body are driven by changes in her hormones. Puberty is triggered when the hypothalamus, a part of the brain strongly associated with control of the endocrine system, begins secreting gonadotropin-releasing hormone (GnRH). It is not clear what triggers the hypothalamus to do this. At first, GnRH is released in bursts several hours apart at night. Gradually, these bursts become longer and stronger until they occur during both day and night. GnRH signals the nearby anterior pituitary to release luteinizing hormone (LH) and follicle-stimulating hormone (FSH). LH and FSH drive most of the physical changes of puberty.

British physician James Tanner (1920–2010) studied the physical changes in girls' breasts during puberty and developed what are called Tanner stages as a way for physicians to evaluate the progress of puberty in individual girls independent of their chronological age. Later, researchers correlated other physical changes in puberty, such as the development of body hair, with Tanner stages. Normal puberty, regardless of how early or late it begins, follows these stages in sequence. Menstruation can begin at any stage except stage 1. The time periods below refer to girls in Western developed countries.

- Stage 1: Puberty has not begun. The nipple of the breast is only barely raised above the chest. The girl has not developed any pubic or underarm hair.
- Stage 2: This is called the breast budding stage. The nipple begins to be raised above the level of the chest. A small amount of light hair starts to grow in the pubic area. This stage occurs roughly between 10.5 and 12.9 years of age. About 10% of girls begin to menstruate in this stage.
- Stage 3: The breasts increase in size, and the colored area around the nipple (the areola) expands. Pubic hair becomes denser, darker, and coarser. Underarm hair is present. This stage generally occurs between ages 11.3 and 13.5 years. By this time, about 30% of girls have had their first menstrual period, technically called menarche.
- Stage 4: The breasts increase in size, and the nipple and areola project outward from the breast. Pubic hair is coarse and curly and covers an increasingly large area. This stage usually occurs between ages 11.8 and 14.0 years. By the end of stage 4, about 90% of girls will have had their first period.
- Stage 5: The breasts take on their final adult size and shape. Pubic hair is coarse, curly, and covers the area it will continue to cover in adulthood. This stage usually occurs between ages 13.3 and 15.5 years, and almost all girls have begun to menstruate by the end of stage 5.

Girls usually begin to menstruate about 2.5 years after their breasts begin to develop, usually around 12.5 years, but in looking at the average ages for the various stages, it is clear that normal, healthy girls of the same age can be in substantially different stages of puberty. This happens because multiple factors affect the timing of puberty, including race, genetics, and body weight. Hispanic and Black girls often begin puberty earlier than Asian and Caucasian girls. If a girl's mother began puberty earlier or later than average, the girl is likely to follow the same pattern.

In the 1850s, the average age to start menstruating in the developed world was around 15. The age has gradually decreased. Researchers believe this is because of better nutrition. Overweight girls are more likely to begin puberty earlier. Thin or underweight girls are likely to begin puberty a bit later than average. Stress, trauma, an extended period of poor nutrition or calorie restriction, and illness can also delay menstruation.

Other changes also occur in puberty that are not directly related to maturation of the reproductive system. Girls undergo a growth spurt of 2 in (5 cm) or more per year with an average total increase in height of 10 in (25 cm) and a weight gain of gain 40–50 lb (18–23 kg). This growth spurt usually stops around age 15 or 16. In addition, an increased percentage of the body becomes fat, and the distribution of fat changes. Breasts enlarge, hips widen, thighs thicken, and the waist becomes better defined. All this is nature's way of preparing a woman's body for the physical demands of pregnancy.

LH and FSH released by the anterior pituitary are the primary hormones responsible for the physical changes that occur during puberty. LH acts on cells in the ovaries to cause them to produce estrogen. Estrogen circulates through the body and is responsible for the development of secondary sex characteristics such as the enlargement of breast tissue.

FSH works directly on the follicles of the ovary. A female is born with all the eggs in her ovaries that she will ever have. These eggs are contained in saclike follicles, but they are not mature. FSH helps the eggs to mature. Eventually, one mature egg (or occasionally two with nonidentical twins) will be released during the menstrual cycle. The role of LH and FSH as the main controllers of the menstrual cycle is discussed in question 15.

Although the development of secondary sex characteristics and the start of menstruation are the most visible changes that occur during puberty, other hormones also play a less visible role. Weak androgens (male hormones) released by the adrenal cortex are mainly responsible for the growth of pubic and body hair. They are also associated with the change in body odor that comes with puberty and with acne that some girls develop. An increase in growth hormone causes the rapid gain in height that occurs during puberty. Other hormones such as insulin and thyroid hormone play a role in the changes in metabolism that result in weight gain and redistribution of body fat.

14. What concerns do girls have about puberty?

Puberty is often a confusing time of up-and-down emotions and physical changes. During puberty, a need for more independence from family develops and concern about friends' opinions and fitting in with a group of peers grows. Interest in the opposite sex increases. Girls (and boys too) are uneasy about the changes happening to their bodies and are quick to compare themselves to other kids of their age. This can lead to teasing and bullying of girls in whom the changes of puberty arrive unusually early or unusually late.

Overwhelmingly, the changes girls experience in puberty as described in question 13 are normal, necessary, and healthy changes. Yet because normal puberty can begin as early as age 8 or as late as age 14, girls of the same age are often in different stages of development, so their bodies will look quite different. Girls are sometimes confused and embarrassed by how their body has changed. This is especially true if no one has prepared them for what to expect and assured them that other girls are going through the same physical changes and emotional reactions.

Some areas of common concern are as follows:

- Breast development. Breast budding, where the nipple lifts above the level of the chest, can begin as young as age 8 or as late as age 13. This is controlled by hormonal changes, but the timing is dependent on three main factors: race/ethnicity, weight, and genetics. Black and Hispanic girls tend to go through puberty earlier than white or Asian girls. Overweight girls also tend to develop breasts earlier, as do those girls whose mothers were early developers. There is also some evidence that certain endocrine disruptors (see question 38) may accelerate the start of puberty. Whether breasts develop early or late, the time when they appear has no effect on their final size or shape.
- Hair and skin. Hormonal changes lead to changes in hair, skin, and body odor. Hair growth is driven by small amounts of androgens made in the adrenal gland in females and by increasing levels of estrogen. About 15% of girls develop light, soft pubic hair even before they develop breasts. As girls mature into women, it is normal for pubic hair to becomes coarse, curly, and cover an increased area.

  Androgens also drive the growth of underarm and leg hair that can be a source of embarrassment, especially for girls with dark hair and light skin. Some girls develop acne. This has nothing to do with hygiene. Acne is stimulated by androgen hormones. Because boys make 20 times more androgens than girls, they tend to have more frequent and severe problems with acne. Severe acne can be treated medically by a dermatologist.
- Menstruation. This is the area of greatest concern for girls going through puberty. (See question 15 for information on the menstrual cycle.) Most girls have their first period about 2.5 years after they develop breast buds. This means a few 10-year-olds have started

menstruating and a few 15-year-olds have not. Menstruation in girls who participate in athletically demanding activities such as figure skating, gymnastics, and ballet where weight control is important may be even more delayed.

The start of menstruation is unpredictable. Girls understandably worry about being embarrassed if they are caught unprepared and do not have access to the pads or tampons they need to manage their menstrual flow. Periods tend to be irregular in the first few years and are sometimes accompanied by unpleasant cramps, complicating their management. Talking to a sympathetic adult woman and understanding what to expect and how to use menstrual supplies can reduce worries about menstruation.

- Mental and emotional health. Bursts of hormones can push emotions to extremes and create unpredictable mood swings during puberty. Insecurity can transform small misunderstandings into major issues. Friendship groups break up and reform. Body comparisons can become a source of hurt. Many girls and boys going through puberty become more impulsive and willing to take risks and experiment with drugs, alcohol, cigarettes, and other off-limit activities. In addition to sex hormones triggering physical emotional and changes during puberty, sleep cycles regulated by the hormone melatonin (see question 32) shift so that it becomes harder to fall asleep early. This often leaves teens grouchy and sleep deprived.

As girls change into women, they become more interested in boys. Interest in dating leads to challenges of navigating new social situations. At this time, some girls find that they are attracted to other girls or women, which creates even more emotional stress. Virtually everyone, no matter how popular or secure appearing, goes through an unsettling period of figuring out how to handle new sexual feelings. A sympathetic adult can ease the path to self-understanding as can online information from reliable organizations listed in the resource section of this book.

15. How do hormones regulate the menstrual cycle?

The menstrual cycle is an approximately monthly cycle directly controlled by four hormones: luteinizing hormone (LH), follicle-stimulating hormone (FSH), estrogen, and progesterone. It begins at puberty and continues until menopause in women who are not pregnant. Menopause usually occurs between ages 45 and 55. The purpose of the menstrual cycle is to prepare a woman's body for pregnancy. If no pregnancy occurs, each month the lining of the uterus is shed causing the woman to bleed from the vagina (menstruate), and then the cycle repeats.

Girls can begin menstruating at any time between ages 9 and 15, although most begin around ages 12–13. Bleeding is sometimes referred to as "having the monthlies" or "on my period." The average menstrual cycle lasts 28 days. The first year or two, or sometimes even longer, the length of the cycle is often irregular. Once the cycle stabilizes, it can be as short as 21 days or as long as 35 days and still be considered normal. Likewise, most girls menstruate for 3–5 days, but the range of normal bleeding is from 2–7 days. Some girls hesitate to do physical activities such as swimming or other sports when they are menstruating. There is no health reason to stop these activities so long as the girl uses appropriate menstrual supplies.

The menstrual cycle is divided into three parts. The following description is based on a 28-day cycle. The start of the menstrual cycle is called the follicular phase. It begins on the first day that a woman bleeds. At the start of the follicular phase, estrogen and progesterone levels are at their lowest. Low hormone levels signal the hypothalamus in the brain to stimulate the anterior pituitary to release LH and FSH. These hormones travel though the bloodstream and act on the ovaries to increase the production of estrogen. Estrogen starts the maturation of multiple eggs in an ovary.

A woman has two ovaries, one on either side of her body. The ovaries contain between one and two million eggs at birth. Every egg is encased in its own follicle, a sac made of a single layer of cells. At birth, the woman has all the eggs she will ever have; she can never make more. Over time, most of the eggs die and are absorbed by the ovary. At puberty, between 300,000 and 400,000 eggs remain. Of these, only one (occasionally two for nonidentical twins) is released from one of the ovaries during each menstrual cycle. Only between 400 and 500 eggs out of the millions of eggs a girl was born with will mature, be released from the ovary, and have the potential to be fertilized and develop into a baby.

The start of menstruation and the follicular phase is often accompanied by uterine cramps. These are thought to be caused by proteins called prostaglandins that stimulate the uterus to contract so that it can shed its lining. Over-the-counter pain medications containing ibuprofen or naproxen, when taken as directed, often help to relieve discomfort from menstrual cramps.

During the first 5 days of the follicular phase, multiple eggs start to mature, but between days 5 and 8, one follicle becomes dominant and produces more estrogen than all the others. The egg in this follicle continues to mature while the others stop growing and gradually are reabsorbed by the ovary. The follicular phase lasts on average for 14 days.

The next phase, the ovulatory phase, is very brief. It occurs at day 14, or the midpoint of the cycle regardless of how long or short the cycle is. A quick increase in LH from the anterior pituitary causes the dominant follicle to burst and release the mature egg. This event is called ovulation. The released egg is then swept into the fallopian tube, which leads to the uterus. Fertilization occurs in the fallopian tube. The egg can live for only about 24 hours after it leaves the ovary. However, a man's sperm can live in the uterus or fallopian tube for up to five days, so a woman is most likely to get pregnant if she has sex up to five days *before* or two days after ovulation.

The final phase of the menstrual cycle is the luteal phase, which lasts about another 14 days. Once the follicle releases the egg, it transforms into a body called the corpus luteum and begins to produce progesterone. Progesterone acts on the lining of the uterus (the endometrium) to stimulate the growth of blood vessels that will bring nutrients to a fertilized egg. Progesterone makes the uterine lining thicken and inhibits muscular contractions to allow an egg to implant. Pregnancy begins once the fertilized egg has implanted in the uterus wall. The corpus luteum will continue to produce progesterone to maintain the pregnancy until the placenta has formed and can take over progesterone production. If the egg has not been fertilized, the corpus luteum stops producing progesterone, and about two weeks after ovulation, the uterus sheds its lining, and the woman menstruates.

For a few years following a girl's first period, menstrual cycles tend to be irregular. Although this may be a nuisance or a worry, it is normal. Most girls settle into a fairly regular cycle by the time they graduate from high school. Nevertheless, life events such as stress, trauma, illness, changes in exercise, severe dieting, and pregnancy can cause missed or irregular periods. If a woman has been menstruating regularly and then stops for 90 days or three cycles, she should see a doctor. She could be pregnant or have developed a condition such as pelvic inflammatory disease (a sexually transmitted infection) or, rarely, have some type of hormonal imbalance (see question 17).

16. What roles do hormones play in premenstrual syndrome (PMS)?

Premenstrual syndrome (PMS) is a set of physical, emotional, and behavioral changes that occur in as many as 75% of women a few days before their period begins each month. The type and severity of symptoms vary widely among women and can change in the same woman from month to month and as a woman ages. PMS symptoms are thought to be brought on by changes in hormone levels during the menstrual cycle and especially by declining levels of estrogen and progesterone in the days before menstruation begins. Symptoms usually disappear by the fourth day of menstruation and often earlier when estrogen levels begin to increase.

Common physical symptoms of PMS include breast soreness, water retention resulting in weight gain, swollen hands and feet, abdominal bloating, constipation or diarrhea, headache, joint and muscle aches, acne outbreaks, and unusual fatigue. Emotional and behavioral symptoms include depression, anxiety, irritability, increased mood swings, angry outbursts, crying spells, insomnia, poor concentration, changes in appetite, increased food cravings, social withdrawal, and changes in sexual desire. PMS can also worsen health problems that are already present such as depression, anxiety, migraines, seizure disorders, asthma, and allergies. Few women experience all these symptoms. Some experience none, or the symptoms are a minor inconvenience. For others, PMS symptoms are severe enough to disrupt the woman's daily activities.

For a woman to be diagnosed with PMS, symptoms must be present at some time during the five days before her period begins. The symptoms must end within four days of her period starting. Symptoms must be severe enough to interfere with some aspect of the woman's normal activities and occur in at least three consecutive menstrual cycles.

According to the American College of Obstetricians and Gynecologists (ACOG), mild and moderate symptoms of PMS can be lessened by changes in diet and exercise. Regular aerobic exercise such as brisk walking, biking, running, cycling, and swimming can improve symptoms, but the exercise must be done regularly, not just on the days when PMS symptoms appear. Relaxation exercises, meditation, yoga, and massage therapy can reduce stress and also lessen symptoms. A diet high in foods made with whole grains, calcium-rich foods such as milk and yogurt, and foods low in sugars and fats is not only healthy but can lessen PMS symptoms. Avoiding caffeine and alcohol and getting at least eight hours of sleep are also helpful.

Many dietary supplements are advertised to reduce or eliminate PMS symptoms. The only supplements suggested by the ACOG are 1,200 mg of calcium daily (especially for teenage girls who usually do not get enough calcium through diet) and magnesium supplements, which may reduce water retention and bloating. Other supplements that have been studied with inconclusive results include vitamin B6, vitamin D, vitamin E, and folic acid (a B vitamin). These may be helpful only if a woman is deficient in these vitamins. Over-the-counter pain medicines containing ibuprofen or naproxen may help to relieve headache and soreness.

Up to 5% of menstruating women have such severe PMS symptoms that they may be diagnosed by a doctor as having premenstrual dysphoric disorder (PMDD). Women with PMDD usually have extreme and prolonged emotional and behavioral changes such as deep depression, suicidal thoughts, panic attacks, and excessive anger toward others in the week or so before their period begins. PMDD is most common in women who have already been diagnosed with depression or anxiety. Women with PMDD symptoms need to see a doctor who can treat their symptoms with prescription drugs.

17. What are the hormonal causes of abnormal periods?

The menstrual cycle is ultimately controlled by the hormones estrogen and progesterone. These hormones are the end products of a chain of interactions known as the hypothalamic-pituitary-ovarian axis. Menstrual periods can be abnormal if any part of the chain functions incorrectly. The hypothalamus produces gonadotropin-releasing hormone (GnRH). GnRH stimulates the anterior pituitary to secrete luteinizing hormone (LH) and follicle-stimulating hormone (FSH). (For more on these hormones, see question 15.) LH and FSH travel through the body and stimulate the female reproductive organs to produce estrogen and progesterone that regulate the menstrual cycle.

Irregular periods, technically called oligomenorrhea, are normal for girls during the first two or three years after they begin to menstruate. When a girl reaches puberty, the hypothalamic-pituitary-ovarian axis is often immature. Researchers do not know exactly why this happens, but if any part of the system is out of balance, monthly periods may be skipped. In addition to skipping periods, menstrual cycles may vary in length. This is not usually a medical problem unless periods are missed for three or more consecutive months. The cycle becomes more regular as girls mature.

Some girls experience heavy menstrual bleeding instead of missed periods. Heavy bleeding is defined as bleeding that lasts more than seven days, bleeding blood clots larger than a quarter, or bleeding through one or more tampons or pads every hour or two for several hours.

Heavy menstrual bleeding has several hormonal causes. Immaturity of the hypothalamic-pituitary-ovarian axis is one of the most common causes in girls who have just started to menstruate and whose periods are irregular. This condition can occur if not enough FSH is released to cause ovulation (see question 15). The follicle may begin to mature but does not complete maturation and does not rupture and release an egg. Without the release of an egg, the corpus luteum, which develops from a ruptured follicle, does not form. The corpus luteum produces progesterone. Without adequate progesterone, the lining of the uterus thickens somewhat but not enough to be shed. When it is finally shed in another cycle, bleeding can be heavy, or the blood may contain clots.

The thyroid gland located in the neck controls many basic metabolic functions (see question 28). An underactive thyroid (hypothyroidism) can cause heavy menstrual bleeding. Paradoxically, an underactive thyroid can also cause irregular periods or the absence of periods for three or more months (technically called amenorrhea). The reasons for this are complex. The hypothalamus releases thyrotropin-releasing hormone (TRH). TRH stimulates the anterior pituitary to release thyroid-stimulating hormone (TSH). TSH triggers the thyroid to produce thyroid hormones.

The production of thyroid hormones is controlled by a negative feedback loop. The amount of thyroid hormone in the blood is continuously monitored by sensors in the hypothalamus. If the thyroid is underactive and does not produce enough hormone, the hypothalamus keeps pouring out TRH. High levels of TRH stimulate the production of another hormone, prolactin, by the pituitary. Prolactin is associated with milk production in new mothers. It also suppresses the production of estrogen by the ovaries, so that ovulation does not occur or occurs only irregularly, causing skipped or absent periods.

A severely overactive thyroid (hyperthyroidism) can also cause absent or skipped periods. This occurs because an excess of thyroid hormone sets off a chain of events that results in a protein that binds with estrogen so that it is not available to act on the follicle. Inadequate estrogen prevents ovulation, which results in skipped or absent periods. The amount of thyroid hormone in the blood can be measured with a simple blood test. Determining whether abnormal thyroid hormone values are the cause of menstrual problems, however, requires additional testing. Both hypo- and hyperthyroidism can be successfully treated.

Polycystic ovary syndrome (PCOS) is another hormonal cause of abnormal periods. PCOS shows up most often during puberty. PCOS is a metabolic disorder of genetic origin in which the woman makes too many androgens (male hormones). This causes the follicles in the ovary to become fluid-filled cysts that fail to release mature eggs. Women with this condition have either infrequent or absent periods. They may also be overweight and have heavy hair growth. The disorder makes it more likely that they will develop type 2 diabetes (see question 35). The condition can be diagnosed by measuring the amount of androgens in the blood and taking an ultrasound of the ovaries to see if cysts are present.

Many other nonhormonal conditions also cause missed or abnormal periods. These include stress (extremely common), certain steroid drugs, blood-thinning drugs, bleeding disorders, eating disorders (especially anorexia nervosa), excessive weight gain, going off hormonal birth control, and almost any serious illness.

18. How does hormonal birth control work?

Most American and European women will use some type of hormonal birth control at some point in their lives. Hormonal birth control works by introducing female hormones into the body to prevent ovulation. If no egg is released from the ovary, conception cannot happen. Hormonal birth control also causes the mucus in the cervix to thicken, making it harder for sperm to reach the uterus. Most hormonal birth control methods contain both estrogen and progestin, a synthetic form of progesterone. There are also a few forms of hormonal birth control that contain only progestin. All hormonal birth control require a prescription from a doctor and must be used exactly as prescribed to prevent pregnancy.

The advantage of all hormonal birth control methods is that they are highly effective. When used perfectly, fewer than 1 in 100 women will become pregnant during the first year of use. When used typically, meaning a pill is occasionally forgotten or a vaginal ring is not inserted in a timely way, about 9 out of 100 women become pregnant during the first year of use. Aside from preventing conception, hormonal birth control has other advantages. It often causes periods to be shorter and lighter with fewer menstrual cramps. It may improve acne and reduce unwanted hair growth, and studies show that it can decrease the chance of developing uterine, ovarian, or colon cancer.

Hormonal birth control has some risks and potential side effects. Using hormonal birth control slightly increases the risk of deep vein thrombosis, which involves the formation of blood clots in the leg that can break lose and cause heart attack or stroke. The risk is higher in women over age 35 who smoke and who already have risk factors for cardiovascular disease such as high cholesterol, obesity, or high blood pressure. Hormonal birth control also causes side effects in many women, including spotting between periods, breast tenderness, headaches, and nausea. The frequency and intensity of these side effects varies among the different types of hormonal birth control and even among different brands of, for example, contraceptive pills. In addition, no type of hormonal birth control provides protection against sexually transmitted infections.

Contraceptive pills are the most familiar form of hormonal birth control. They are used by about 16% of girls aged 15–19 and by almost one in five women aged 20–29. After age 30, other forms of birth control tend to be preferred. Birth control pills contain estrogen and progestin. Different brands of pills may be taken on different schedules, but all should be taken at the same time each day for maximal protection against pregnancy. A smartphone alarm can be a helpful reminder.

- 21-day pills are taken consecutively for 21 days and then stopped for 7 days, during which time the woman menstruates.
- 28-day pills are taken for 28 days, but only the first 21 pills (or in some brands the first 24 pills) contain hormones. The remainder do not, and while taking the hormone-free pills, the woman menstruates.
- 90-day pills are taken consecutively for 90 days. The last 7 pills contain no hormones, and the woman menstruates every three months while taking the hormone-free pills.
- 365-day pills are taken year-round. The woman may have very light periods or none at all.
- Minipills are progestin-only pills. They prevent pregnancy by thickening the mucus of the cervix to prevent sperm from reaching the uterus and thinning the uterine lining so that a fertilized egg cannot implant. They suppress ovulation, although not as completely as pills that contain both estrogen and progestin. Minipills are safe to take when breastfeeding. They may be a better choice for women over age 35 and those with high blood pressure, a history of blood clots, or who are taking certain medications.

Contraceptive pills are not the only form of hormonal birth control. Vaginal rings are flexible plastic rings that contain estrogen and progestin. They must be prescribed by a doctor but are inserted by the woman. The ring remains in place for 21 days. During this time, the hormones in the ring are absorbed through the walls of the vagina. On day 22, the woman removes the ring. After seven days, during which time she menstruates, she inserts a new ring and repeats the cycle. The advantage of the ring is that once it is in place, it can be forgotten for 21 days. The woman does not have to remember to take a pill every day. Side effects of the vaginal ring are the same as for the pill, but they may also cause increased vaginal discharge.

Contraceptive skin patches are another form hormonal birth control. They can be worn on the upper arm, back, buttocks, or abdomen. The patch is worn continuously for 21 days. During this time estrogen and progestin are absorbed through the skin. After 21 days, the patch is removed, and the woman menstruates. In seven days, she applies a new patch. Skin patches have generally minor side effects, although in some women, they may cause skin irritation.

The contraceptive shot is an injection that contains only progestin. It is given every three months. Advantages are that once the woman has the shot, she does not have to be concerned about birth control for three months. In addition, she may have no or very light periods and little menstrual cramping. One disadvantage is the need to return to a health care provider every three months for another shot. Depending on insurance coverage, this may be an added cost. The shot also causes irregular spotting in some women. Once the shot is discontinued, it takes some women a few months to return to a regular cycle. Long-term use of the shot also causes bone loss.

A contraceptive implant is the most effective form of birth control. Implants are used by only 3.5% of women aged 15–44. The implant is inserted in the arm and provides get-it-and-forget-it contraception for three years. Side effects are the same as for other forms of hormonal birth control but sometimes may be more extreme. About 20% of women choose to have their implant removed because of side effects.

An intrauterine device (IUD) is a T-shaped device that is placed in the uterus by a health care provider. There are two types, one made of copper that contains no hormones and another that contains progestin. Once inserted, a copper IUD can prevent conception for up to 10 years. Progestin-containing IUDs are effective for 3–5 years. Advantages are that once in place, birth control is continuous without any effort from the woman, and she continues to have her normal periods. Once removed, the woman can quickly become pregnant if she wants a pregnancy. Disadvantages are that an IUD may be difficult to insert into a woman who has not had a baby and that it must be removed by a health care provider should the woman wish to become pregnant. In addition, intense cramping may follow insertion. Rarely is the IUD expelled and rarely does insertion cause infection.

A sexually active woman who uses no birth control has an 85% chance of becoming pregnant within one year. All hormonal birth control methods are more effective than any barrier method, such as male or female condoms, spermicidal foam, or the diaphragm. The choice of birth control method depends on the woman's ability to use the method consistently and correctly, the side effects she experiences, and her partner's willingness to cooperate in preventing conception. Most women try several types of birth control throughout their reproductive years either because they find the side effects of a specific type unacceptable or because their lifestyle changes as they age, and this changes the factors they consider most important in choosing a birth control method.

19. How do pregnancy tests work?

How can you tell if you are pregnant? If you lived in ancient Egypt, you would urinate for several days on wheat or barley seeds. If the seeds sprouted, you were pregnant. If they didn't, you were not. This sounds like an old wives' tale, but in 1963, scientists tested this method and found that it was 70% accurate.

Fast-forward to 1927. Two German scientists, Selmar Aschheim (1878–1965) and Bernhard Zondek (1891–1966), discovered that if a pregnant woman's urine was injected into an immature female mouse, the mouse would ovulate even though she was immature. If nothing happened, the woman was not pregnant. Getting the answer took five days, but the results were more than 98% accurate. The mice had to be killed and dissected to determine if they had ovulated, so the cost in terms of mice and time was high, and the test was not often done.

American scientist Maurice Friedman (1903–1991) substituted rabbits for mice in 1931. A rabbit was easier to inject, gave results in one day, but still had to be killed. To solve this problem, British scientist Lancelot Hogben (1885–1975) found that the urine of pregnant women caused frogs to lay eggs. Since the eggs were laid outside the body, the frogs did not need to be killed, and they were a lot less expensive than rabbits. Frogs were used until the early 1970s, and pregnancy testing was done only when there was a medical need to know early on if a woman was pregnant.

The magic chemical in pregnant women's urine that causes changes in mice, rabbits, and frogs is the hormone human chorionic gonadotropin (hCG), which is removed from the body in urine. Once an egg is released from the ovary, the follicle, or sac the egg matured in, becomes a structure called the corpus luteum. The corpus luteum begins producing the hormone progesterone, which is essential for changing the uterine lining to support a pregnancy. If fertilization does not occur, the corpus luteum stops progesterone production, and the lining is shed (menstruation). However, if a fertilized egg implants in the uterus wall, cells surrounding the embryo immediately begin secreting hCG. hCG tells the corpus luteum to keep making progesterone until the placenta is developed enough to take over its production for the remainder of the pregnancy. The amount of hCG doubles about every 48 hours. Levels peak at between 8 and 11 weeks of pregnancy. One theory is that hCG causes or contributes to the morning sickness many women experience early in pregnancy.

Modern blood and urine pregnancy tests were developed in the early 1970s. Initially, these test were complicated and had to be done in a doctor's office. The results often took several hours, and the tests usually were not performed until well after a woman had missed her menstrual period. This changed in 1978, when an early pregnancy test that could be done by the woman herself at home became available in the United States. The tests are sold in pharmacies and supermarkets at a reasonable cost and without a prescription.

Home pregnancy tests are antibody-based tests. Antibodies are part of the immune system. Most often they stick to foreign bacteria and viruses to destroy them and keep us healthy. However, for a pregnancy test, researchers modified antibodies against hCG and attached them to sheep blood. When a woman is pregnant, the hCG antibodies on the sheep blood attach to the hCG in her urine. This make the blood clump in a specific pattern that indicates the woman is pregnant. No clumping meant no pregnancy.

In 1988, a simplified antibody-based home pregnancy test was developed that is still used today. Although the exact instructions for using and interpreting different brands of tests vary, all home tests work on the same principle. They use a stick that contains a line of hCG antibodies and a control line. When exposed to a pregnant woman's urine, the antibodies latch on to hCG in the urine, but instead of causing blood to clump, the antibody-hCG complex within minutes activates a colored dye. The presence of a colored line indicates that the woman is pregnant. If no hCG is present, the colored line does not appear, and the woman is not pregnant. Modern tests are sensitive enough to detect the presence of hCG between 10 and 14 days after conception. When used correctly, they are 99% accurate.

20. What hormonal changes occur during pregnancy and birth?

When a woman becomes pregnant, there are many external signs. Her abdomen bulges, her breasts increase in size, and her food preferences may change. But what are the internal changes to her body that bring about these external changes? Pregnancy and giving birth cause a cascade of hormonal changes. The quantities of luteinizing hormone (LH) and follicle-stimulating hormone (FSH), the hormones that control the menstrual cycle and ovulation, are so low during pregnancy as to effectively be inactive. This prevents conception and menstruation once a woman is pregnant. The familiar female hormones estrogen and progesterone take on new roles, while other hormones normally made in small quantities take on major roles during pregnancy and birth.

- Human chorionic gonadotropin (hCG) is the hormone that announces that a woman is pregnant. It is the substance tested for by pregnancy tests (see question 19). hCG is made very early in pregnancy by cells that surround the developing embryo. It can be detected by a correctly used home pregnancy test as early as 10–14 days after conception. hCG is most active during the first trimester. It triggers the production of estrogen and progesterone and may be partially responsible for morning sickness.
- Human placental lactogen (HPL) is produced beginning around the second week of pregnancy and can be detected by a blood test by week six. HPL primarily works to ensure that the fetus gets adequate nutrition. It helps the body break down fats and makes the body more resistant to insulin (see question 34) so that less glucose (sugar) enters the mother's cells and more is available to nourish the fetus. It also plays a role in stimulating the milk glands in the breast to prepare for nursing a newborn.
- Estrogen is normally made by the ovaries, but during pregnancy, the presence of hCG also triggers its production by the placenta. Women make large amounts of estrogen during pregnancy. This hormone helps the uterus grow to accommodate the growing fetus. It increases the growth of blood vessels in the placenta and plays a role in maturation of the fetus. Estrogen begins increasing early in the first trimester. This increase may play a role in morning sickness and mood swings. Estrogen levels peak around week 32 of pregnancy.
- In pregnancy, progesterone is first produced by the corpus luteum and then by the placenta. Progesterone begins to increase early in the first trimester. It helps to build and maintain the lining of the uterus, prevents the uterus from contracting, and increases blood supply to the breasts, which stimulates their growth. Progesterone may play a role in mood swings and fatigue.
- Relaxin is a hormone produced very early in pregnancy by the corpus luteum to help prepare the uterine lining for implantation. It

also helps prevent the uterus from contracting. Later in pregnancy, relaxin is made by the placenta. It is best known for relaxing the muscles, ligaments, and joints in preparation for labor and delivery.

• Oxytocin is secreted from the posterior pituitary. It is present throughout pregnancy, but it is most active in the third trimester and after birth. It causes the membranes around the fetus to break and the uterus to contract during labor. After the baby is born, oxytocin helps the uterus expel the placenta. It also promotes bonding between mother and baby. Synthetic oxytocin called Pitocin is sometimes given to a woman to start labor or to one whose contractions during labor are weak.

• Prolactin is produced by the anterior pituitary. It causes the breasts to increase in size and the internal development of mammary glands. When a baby nurses, the stimulation from sucking causes the release of more prolactin, which results in additional milk production.

21. How are the baby blues and postpartum depression related to hormonal changes?

Dramatic changes in a woman's hormone balance occur a few days before labor begins and continue after delivery. With so many physical and hormonal changes in a short period, combined with the stress and sleep deprivation of having a new baby, it is not surprising that a woman's mood is affected. The hormonal and emotional factors combine to produce a condition called the baby blues in almost all women shortly after they have given birth. Women with the baby blues cry easily, feel overwhelmed and emotionally fragile, and have frequent mood swings. These feelings generally peak between five and seven days after delivery and then gradually taper off by the end of the second week. Baby blues are normal, but it helps to accept them by understanding why they occur and realizing that they are temporary.

Before labor begins, the hormone relaxin is secreted by the placenta. This hormone helps soften the cervix and relax the ligaments in the pelvis to make delivery easier. It also helps the membranes surrounding the baby rupture, causing a woman's water to break. It can take several months after the birth for these ligaments to tighten up again. This can occasionally affect a woman's sense of balance and stability.

Once labor starts, a woman's body is flooded with endorphins. These are chemicals that act on receptors in the brain to reduce pain, produce feelings of euphoria, and alter the perception of time. Endorphins are some of the same chemicals that help to activate what marathon runners call a runner's high. After delivery, the level of endorphins quickly drops, and those good feelings are lost. This may contribute to the emotional state known as the baby blues.

Throughout pregnancy, estrogen levels rise steadily to the point where they can be up to 100 times higher than before pregnancy. Estrogen levels generally peak around week 32 of pregnancy. Shortly after delivery, estrogen levels start to drop, although not as fast as progesterone levels. The decrease in estrogen is thought to play a role in both mood swings and a feeling of fatigue, discouragement, and uncertainty that may occur in the weeks after delivery.

From very early in pregnancy, the placenta has been pumping out progesterone to prevent miscarriage and support the pregnancy in other ways. Soon after the baby is delivered, the placenta detaches from the uterus and is expelled. Without the placenta, progesterone levels abruptly drop to near their prepregnancy levels. Because estrogen levels drop more slowly, there is an imbalance between these hormones.

The imbalance between estrogen and progesterone is thought to play a role in the development of thyroid gland inflammation, which occurs in up to 10% of women within several months after delivery. The thyroid controls many aspects of metabolism (see questions 28 and 29). A postpartum underactive thyroid (hypothyroidism) is most common. Too little thyroid hormone can cause fatigue, depression, increased sensitivity to cold, and weight gain. Postpartum hypothyroidism can last for several months and usually clears up on its own. Too much thyroid hormone (hyperthyroidism) is less common. It can cause anxiety, irritability, insomnia, and increased sensitivity to heat. Symptoms of both hyper- and hypothyroidism are often incorrectly thought to be caused by the stress of caring for a new baby, so thyroid hormone imbalances often go undiagnosed.

Other hormonal changes also occur with labor and delivery. To strengthen uterine contractions during labor, the body produces the hormone oxytocin. Oxytocin production continues after delivery when it acts in two ways. It encourages mother-baby bonding (oxytocin is sometimes called the "love hormone"), and it stimulates the movement of milk into the mammary glands. Milk production is controlled by another hormone, prolactin. Prolactin is present during pregnancy, but its actions are suppressed by high levels of estrogen. Once estrogen decreases, milk production increases, which is why it may take a few days for a woman's milk to come in.

The baby blues are considered normal and need no treatment. In some women, however, these feelings of being overwhelmed, unable to cope, constantly tired, and unhappy do not fade, but deepen and become postpartum depression (PPD). PPD is a medical problem that should be treated. Women with PPD may have frequent crying jags, intense sadness, insomnia, irritability, feelings of worthlessness, and suicidal thoughts. They may become hypervigilant and overly concerned about their baby's safety, sometimes to the point of not letting anyone else handle the baby. Racing thoughts may prevent them from sleeping. This condition of being hypervigilant and unreasonably worried is sometimes called postpartum anxiety (PPA).

There is no single reason why some women develop PPD or PPA, although isolation, previous episodes of mood disturbances, an abusive relationship, and excessive stress such as financial worries make a woman more susceptible to developing these conditions. PPD and PPA should be brought to the attention of a health care professional, as they can be successfully treated.

One serious mood disorder associated with the postpartum period is postpartum psychosis. Postpartum psychosis is rare, and it is not clear if or how it is related to hormonal changes. It usually begins within a week or two after giving birth, and it is a medical emergency. The new mother may think she sees or hears things that are not there (hallucinations) or develop irrational beliefs (delusions) such as the baby being possessed by an evil spirit. She may have thoughts of harming her baby, paranoia, rapid mood swings, insomnia, and extreme irritability. In short, she has lost her grip on reality (a psychotic break) and needs immediate psychiatric intervention. Getting this intervention falls to the woman's partner and family, as she cannot recognize the danger of her emotional state. There is a 4% infanticide and 5% suicide rate in women with postpartum psychosis. If any doubt exists about the woman's grasp on reality and the safety of her baby or herself, an immediate trip to the emergency room is appropriate.

22. What are the predominantly male sex hormones?

Androgens are sex hormones that promote and maintain male physical characteristics and the male reproductive system. The main male sex hormone is testosterone. It is secreted by the testes (also called testicles or gonads). These two oval organs, each the size of a large grape, are located in the scrotum, a sac that hangs outside the body below the penis. The cortex of the adrenal gland also makes a small amount of testosterone.

The level of testosterone circulating in the body is controlled by a negative feedback loop that connects the hypothalamus, pituitary gland, and testes. The hypothalamus releases gonadotropin-releasing hormone (GnRH). GnRH then stimulates the anterior pituitary to release luteinizing hormone (LH). LH signals Leydig cells in the testes to make testosterone, which is secreted into the blood. When sensors in the hypothalamus determine that too much testosterone is circulating, no more GnRH is released. When testosterone levels fall too low, GnRH release begins again. Two other androgens, androstenedione and dehydroepiandrosterone (DHEA), have only weak direct effects on male characteristics. However, they are important because the body converts them into testosterone, a much more powerful hormone.

Testosterone is responsible for the changes that occur during puberty. Puberty for boys starts on average at age 12, but it is completely normal for it to start earlier or later—anywhere between ages 9 and 14 (see question 23). During puberty, testosterone remodels the male body. The penis and testes enlarge. Hair grows on the face, body, and pubic area. The voice deepens. As boys become men, they grow taller, develop larger and stronger muscles, and make denser, stronger bones. Interest in sex also increases. Adult men continue to need testosterone to support the reproductive system, make mature sperm, maintain their sex drive, and have effective erections. Testosterone helps maintain muscle mass and bone strength. It can also affect mood and energy level.

The amount of testosterone a man makes peaks in his early 20s and begins to decrease significantly around age 35. Conditions such as injury to the testes; infections; HIV/AIDS; chemotherapy; radiation; tumors of the pituitary or hypothalamus; morphine, codeine, and similar opium derivatives; major tranquilizers; and alcoholism can cause low testosterone independent of the natural decline caused by aging. Low testosterone can result in a reduced sex drive and poor or failed erections, low sperm count, loss of strength and muscle mass, weakened bones, and increased body fat.

High levels of natural testosterone are an uncommon problem in men, but when they occur, the cause is often a tumor of the adrenal gland or testicular cancer. Abnormally high testosterone levels can also be caused by taking anabolic steroid drugs (see question 39) or overtreatment with testosterone skin gel or testosterone shots. In the case of testosterone, more is *not* better. Prolonged high levels will cause low sperm counts and impotence. This may seem contradictory, but when the level of testosterone is increased from outside sources such as skin gels, the hypothalamus shuts down production of testosterone in the testes. Without this testosterone, sperm, which are also made in the testes, do not mature. Other side effects of high testosterone can include heart muscle damage, difficulty urinating due to an enlarged prostate, acne, fluid retention, high blood pressure, increased aggression, mood swings, irritability, and impaired judgment.

There is general agreement in the medical community that delayed puberty and low testosterone due to injury or certain medical conditions (e.g., HIV, chemotherapy) are appropriate reasons for using supplemental or replacement testosterone. More controversial is the idea that low testosterone due to natural aging should be treated. Advertising by clinics that treat male sexual problems suggests that treating low testosterone due to aging will restore a man's sex drive and sexual performance, help him lose fat and gain muscle, improve energy level, lift mood, and make him feel younger. These claims are both supported and disproved by various clinical studies and should be viewed skeptically.

One problem with treating low testosterone is that few standards exist for determining what should be considered a low level of testosterone. Testosterone can be measured with a simple blood test, but interpretation of the results depends on several variables. Testosterone production is cyclical, and the hormone is not stored in the body. The level is highest in the morning and the lowest at night, so interpreting test values depends on when a blood sample was taken. In addition, there is little agreement on what value should be considered low at any given age. Finally, there is disagreement over the point at which the benefits of treatment outweigh the risks of creating other health problems for patients.

23. What occurs during puberty in boys?

Puberty is a time of great physical, emotional, social, and hormonal changes. When it begins, a boy is still a child. By the time it ends, his body shape has changed, and he is physically a man capable of fathering a child. Puberty can begin in boys as young as age 9 or as old as age 15 and still be considered normal. On average in the United States, puberty in boys begins between ages 11 and 12 and ends between ages 16 and 19. Boys generally start puberty about two years later than girls of the same age. Normal healthy boys can be the same chronological age and be in vastly different stages of physical maturation. Researchers believe that multiple factors affect the timing of puberty, including genetics, body weight, and nutrition. Genetics appears to have the strongest influence; boys tend to go through puberty at about the same time as their fathers did.

The physical changes in a boy's body are driven by changes in the concentration of male hormones, primarily testosterone. Puberty is triggered when the hypothalamus, a part of the brain strongly associated with control of the endocrine system, begins secreting gonadotropin-releasing hormone (GnRH). It is not clear what triggers the hypothalamus to do this. GnRH is released in bursts one to two hours apart. Gradually, these bursts become longer and stronger. GnRH signals the nearby anterior pituitary gland to release luteinizing hormone (LH) and, to a lesser extent, follicle-stimulating hormone (FSH). Interestingly, LH and FSH stimulate most of the physical changes in both boys and girls, although they work on different tissues in each sex and produce different results.

British physician James Tanner (1920–2010) studied the physical changes in boys' reproductive anatomy during puberty and developed what are called Tanner stages as a way for physicians to evaluate the progress of puberty in individual boys independent of their chronological age. Later, researchers correlated other changes in puberty, such as the development of body hair, with Tanner stages. Regardless of how early or late puberty begins or how fast it progresses, normal puberty always follows these stages in sequence.

- Stage 1: Puberty has not begun. The testes and penis are small. Testicular volume is less than 1.5 mL. Any hair present is soft, light vellus hair ("peach fuzz"). No curly pubic hair is present.
- Stage 2: The testes and scrotum begin to grow, and the scrotum thins and reddens. The penis enlarges but only by a small amount. A few dark, straight pubic hairs appear, usually at the base of the penis. This stage often occurs between ages 9 and 11.
- Stage 3: The testes and scrotum continue to enlarge. The penis becomes longer. Dark, curly pubic hair and underarm hair begin to appear as the result of stimulation by androgens. This stage occurs on average between ages 11 and 12.5 years.
- Stage 4: The testes continue to grow. The penis elongates and becomes thicker. The scrotum enlarges and darkens. Curly, coarse, dark pubic hair increases. On average, this stage occurs between ages 12.5 and 14. Boys begin to have ejaculations. Sperm production occurs early in puberty, so a boy who is having ejaculations may be capable of fathering a child before all the stages of puberty are complete.
- Stage 5: The testes and scrotum reach their final adult size. Testicular volume is more than 13 times greater than in stage 1. The penis reaches its adult size and shape. Pubic hair is coarse, curly, and dense. It covers the area it will continue to cover in adulthood. This stage usually occurs between ages 14 and 18.

The changes described by the Tanner stages occur because of a complex interplay of hormones. The release of LH by the pituitary stimulates Leydig cells in the testes to produce increased amounts of testosterone in a cyclical pattern with the highest amounts released in the morning and the lowest in the evening. During puberty, the body converts a much higher amount of this testosterone into a compound called dihydrotestosterone than occurs during any other stage of life. Dihydrotestosterone is a much stronger, more potent form of testosterone. It acts on many different tissues and directs most of the changes during puberty, including maturation of the male reproductive organs, increase in bone and muscle mass, hair growth, and increased sex drive.

Other changes also occur in puberty that are not directly related to maturation of the reproductive organs. Boys undergo a growth spurt of on average 3 in (7.6 cm) per year for several years. The average American boy will be less than 54.5 in (138.5 cm) tall before puberty and reach a final adult height of 69.1 in (175.4 cm) after going through puberty. This is a theoretical "average" boy, but it demonstrates how quickly boys grow during puberty. In a healthy person, about 80% of final height is determined by genetics, with the remainder determined by nutrition and other environmental factors. Growth in boys slows around age 16, but height usually increases slowly by an inch or two until about age 20. Starting puberty late does not reduce a boy's final height; he simply grows faster than a boy who started puberty early.

Body shape also changes as bones become more dense and muscle mass increases. The body acquires a triangular, wide shoulder-narrow waist shape. Body odor and sweating become more pronounced, and oily skin accompanied by acne is likely to develop because of increased androgen levels. Facial hair usually appears about two years after pubic hair.

The first erection usually occurs once the penis begins to grow toward its adult size. This is soon followed by the first ejaculation. In American boys, the first ejaculation often occurs between ages 12.5 and 14, although there is a great deal of normal variation. Once a boy has erections and can ejaculate, he is capable of causing a pregnancy.

24. What concerns do boys have about puberty?

Puberty can be a confusing time of unstable emotions and awkward physical changes. Friends and their opinions take on more importance, and boys (girls also) are quick to compare themselves to others. Fitting in becomes increasingly important as boys draw away from their families.

Increased testosterone levels are associated with increased aggression and risk-taking behavior. Exploring the boundaries of independence and trying to fit in with peers sometimes leads to inappropriate, tasteless, or dangerous behavior. Add to this an increased interest in sex and socially telegraphed ideas about how a man should act, and puberty can be hard, confusing, and sometimes lonely.

The physical changes that boys go through during puberty (see question 23) are normal, necessary, and healthy changes. Yet because normal puberty can begin as early as age 9 or as late as age 15, boys of the same age are often in different stages of development, so their bodies look quite different. These differences can be a source of embarrassment and bullying, especially for boys who enter puberty late. Boys who play sports such as football or basketball may feel especially disadvantaged by a late puberty and its accompanying late growth spurt.

Most common concerns of boys during puberty are not medical problems. They are normal changes that must be lived through with the knowledge that everyone else is going through similar problems. These concerns are almost always linked to changing hormone levels, and most will disappear on their own with time and maturity. Some common areas of concern include the following:

- Random erections. During puberty and into early adulthood, it is common to experience random, involuntary erections. The stimulus can be almost anything, even something extremely minor. Although they are perfectly normal, involuntary erections can happen at awkward times and be a source of embarrassment. The best option is to try to hide the erection by shielding it behind an object, focusing on something completely nonsexual, and doing nothing to call attention to the situation.

- Wet dreams. Involuntary ejaculations at night are also extremely common. While asleep, boys going through puberty and young adult men will have on average three to five erections every night, each lasting approximately 30 minutes. These can result in nocturnal ejaculations. Wet dreams are caused by hormonal fluctuations during sleep. They are not under conscious control. Eventually as a man ages, they lessen and then stop.

- Breast enlargement. Many boys experience a tender, sometimes painful, lump under one or both nipples. Breast enlargement in men is technically called gynecomastia. It usually occurs early in puberty and is the result of an imbalance between estrogen and testosterone. The condition in puberty is cosmetic and not a medical concern.

Breast enlargement normally disappears on its own, although it may take months and cause embarrassment until it does.

- Sweating and body odor. These both increase due to increasing levels of testosterone. They can be controlled by increased awareness of personal hygiene.
- Acne. Boys are more likely to have severe acne than girls. The cause is not poor hygiene, but increasing levels of testosterone. Acne can be treated with over-the-counter acne products and, in severe cases, prescription medication. Permanent scars can result if the acne is picked at or scratched. Otherwise, the condition generally disappears with age.
- Facial hair. Both pubic and facial hair growth are stimulated by testosterone, but testosterone levels are only one factor that determines how much facial hair a man has. Genetics play a large role in determining the density of a man's beard. Hair and skin color also affect the perception of beard thickness. Facial hair usually appears about two years after pubic hair and will continue to increase and grow coarser until around age 30, so thin facial hair in puberty does not necessarily mean thin facial hair in adulthood.

As boys change into men, their sex drive increases, and they become very interested in girls. Navigating dating and new social situations with girls can be nerve wracking. Virtually everyone, no matter how popular or secure appearing, goes through an unsettling period of figuring out how to handle these new sexual feelings. Boys often brag about sexual experience, ramping up social pressure among their peers to be sexually active. Talk and reality, however, are two different things. A 2019 study by the Institute for Family Studies found that only 39% of high school boys reported having ever had sexual intercourse before graduation.

During puberty, some boys find that they are attracted to other boys or men or that they do not identify with their biological sex. This usually creates huge confusion, self-doubt, emotional stress, and the potential for serious depression. A sympathetic adult can ease the path to self-understanding as can online information from reliable organizations listed in the resource section of this book.

25. What are the hormonal causes of erectile dysfunction?

Erectile dysfunction (ED) occurs when a man cannot have an erection or cannot maintain it long enough for satisfactory sex. All men occasionally have this problem, especially after heavy alcohol or drug use or when very tired, but if ED happens more than occasionally, it can indicate a physical problem or a mental health issue such as depression.

Studies of how many men have ED produce a wide range of numbers depending on how the condition is defined and the culture in which the survey is done. Studies suggest that about one-quarter of men between ages 17 and 40 experience occasional ED, while half of men over age 40 and 60% of men in their 60s have at least mild ED. Other studies have found rates ranging from 3% to 76%, so the real rate is difficult to determine.

Having an erection involves the brain, nerve impulses, muscles, and hormones. All erections start in the brain when a man is sexually stimulated. Once aroused, the brain sends a message to the local nerves of the penis. These nerves then signal the muscles of the penis to relax. This may seem contradictory, but inside the penis are two parallel cylinders called the corpora cavernosa. Each cylinder is filled with spongelike tissue and has an artery supplying it with blood. When the muscles of the penis relax, the arteries in the cylinders widen. This means that they can bring more blood to the penis.

The extra blood fills the spaces within the spongelike tissue until the spaces are full, causing the cylinders to expand. This makes the penis hard. At the same time, veins that carry blood away from the penis are closed down. The penis remains hard until the veins open, blood flows out, and the spongy tissue deflates. This can happen rapidly after ejaculation or gradually if there is no additional stimulation.

Nitric oxide is a chemical made in the body that helps relax and open up blood vessels. An enzyme called oral phosphodiesterase type 5 (PDE5) interferes with the action of nitric oxide. Drugs advertised to treat ED such as sildenafil (Viagra), tadalafil (Cialis), vardenafil (Levitra), and avanafil (Stendra) work by limiting the production of PDE5. This has the effect of increasing the amount of nitric oxide available to open blood vessels and increasing blood flow to the penis so that it hardens. More invasive treatments for ED are available if these drugs do not produce the desired result.

ED has many causes. In younger men, the cause is often, but not always, psychological. Worry about performance, prolonged stress (emotional, economic, professional), relationship conflicts (his partner wants a baby, but he does not), depression, and anxiety can all cause ED in physically health men. On the other hand, ED may be a sign of a physical health issue.

Circulatory system problems are an especially common cause. Artery walls may be thickened and hardened (arteriosclerosis) so that they do not expand enough to allow the corpora cavernosa to receive the volume of blood needed to create an erection. Arteries can also be clogged with fats or damaged by high levels of glucose in the blood, restricting blood flow. Occasionally nerves to the penis may be damaged. Obesity, diabetes, alcoholism, and drug addiction frequently cause or worsen ED.

Abnormal hormone production can also cause ED. Low testosterone levels may prevent some men achieving a satisfactory erection, although no direct relationship between testosterone levels and ED has ever been established. Some studies have found that 40% of men over age 45 have low testosterone; however, there is controversy over how to measure testosterone levels and what values should be considered low (see question 22). Testosterone supplementation is not a magic key to eliminating ED. Only about one-third of men with low testosterone and ED improve when given supplemental testosterone.

Other hormonal causes of ED include too much thyroid hormone (hyperthyroidism) or too little thyroid hormone (hypothyroidism). Thyroid hormone regulates many basic metabolic functions (see question 28). Hypothyroidism most commonly causes depression, low sex drive, fatigue, ED, and delayed ejaculation. Premature ejaculation is more likely to be associated with hyperthyroidism. Thyroid levels can be checked with a simple blood test and corrected with medication.

An uncommon cause of ED is excess production of the hormone prolactin. Prolactin is made in the anterior pituitary. It is best known for promoting milk production in nursing mothers, but men also make this hormone in small amounts. Sometimes small, benign (noncancerous) tumors in the pituitary cause the gland to produce too much prolactin. Prolactin interferes with the production of testosterone and sperm. This decreases sex drive and can cause ED. Once diagnosed, excess prolactin can be successfully treated with drugs.

26. How do hormones influence biological sex, gender identity, and sexual orientation?

What is the difference between biological sex, gender identity, and sexual orientation? Researchers are currently exploring the roles of genetics, hormone exposure during fetal development, and socialization after birth in the development of these complex characteristics. They have found that biological sex, gender identity, and sexual orientation are not always aligned and are likely to develop from different patterns of influences.

A person's biological sex derives from inherited chromosomes (usually XX for females and XY for males). Gender identity is the individual's strongly held internal identification as male, female, or nonbinary. Gender identity is the individual's deep belief about their gender. Gender identity can be the same as or different from the individual's biological sex. Sexual orientation is the pattern of physical and emotional attraction to another person of the same or opposite sex or to both sexes. Some people may be asexual and feel little sexual attraction to either sex.

For the first six weeks after fertilization, all fetuses have tissue that can develop into either female or male reproductive organs. This is true whether the fetal chromosomes are XX or XY. At about seven weeks, genes on the Y chromosome trigger the production of androgens that are converted into testosterone. Testosterone signals the undifferentiated fetal tissue to develop into male reproductive organs, while a second hormone suppresses the development of female reproductive organs. In the absence of early prenatal androgens, the fetus develops physically as female.

The process of sex organ differentiation is complicated, and there are many opportunities for errors and abnormalities to occur. About one in every 1,500–2,000 babies is identified as having a disorder of sexual differentiation (DSD). These individuals were formerly called intersex babies because they show signs of having both male and female reproductive organs, or they have nonstandard sex chromosomes. Researchers are still sorting out why DSDs happen, but they have identified several hormonal reasons. For example, an XX fetus may have a condition called congenital adrenal hyperplasia that causes the adrenal glands to inappropriately produce androgens that partially masculinize the fetus. In other cases, an XY fetus may develop female organs because of a condition called androgen insensitivity syndrome. In other words, the fetus produces androgens, but the target tissue fails to respond to them.

Chromosomal irregularities are also possible. People with Klinefelter's syndrome, for example, have an extra X chromosome (XXY). These individuals are assigned male at birth, but the extra X chromosome interferes with the production of testosterone. They may need testosterone supplements and require assistive reproductive techniques such as in vitro fertilization to have children. Other nonstandard chromosomal combinations include females with one X chromosome (XO) or with three X chromosomes (XXX). Some individuals have one or two X chromosomes but also incomplete bits of Y chromosome.

In the past, babies born with ambiguous sex organs were often assigned by the doctor to a biological sex, and surgery was promptly performed to make the sex organs conform to the assigned sex. Today, the trend is to allow these individuals to keep their ambiguous sex organs intact until they are old enough to develop gender identity and then offer surgery to make their body conform to their internal identity.

The formation of gender identity is difficult to research and is hotly debated. Identical twin studies suggest that genes play only a minor role in its formation. Evidence exists both for and against the role of prenatal hormones in the development of gender identity. The strongest evidence suggests that gender identity is at least partially formed by the effect of prenatal sex hormones on the organization and function of the developing brain. However, the reliability of this research is limited by small sample size, and findings are open to a variety of interpretations.

One recent study found that prenatal exposure of females to androgens did not change the amount of time they spent playing with other girls. However, girls who were exposed to prenatal androgens spent significantly more time in traditionally "male" activities such as building things, playing with cars, and watching sports, even though almost all the androgen-exposed girls in the study had female gender identity. This study did not consider socialization or environmental factors that could affect gender identity development. People whose biological sex does not match their gender identity are considered to have gender dysphoria. Individuals in this situation may seek psychological and medical help to resolve this disparity (see question 27).

Sexual orientation may or may not align with biological sex and/or gender identity. Sexual orientation exists along a continuum from asexual to strictly heterosexual to bisexual to strictly homosexual. Research strongly suggests that genes and hormones are major factors in determining an individual's sexual orientation. However, researchers also have found that sexual orientation is more complex than just the presence or absence of androgens. There is significant overlap in the amount of androgens found in strictly heterosexual men with low androgen levels and strictly heterosexual women with high androgen levels (see case illustration 5). One thought is that sexual orientation may be at least partially regulated by the early balance between androgens and estrogens in both sexes. Something researchers do agree on is that sexual orientation is a biological construct, not a choice. There is no evidence that socialization, societal disapproval, or any type of therapy will change an individual's sexual orientation.

27. How are hormones used to help transgender people transition?

When an individual's assigned biological sex as male or female is different from their gender identity (the strong internal sense of being male, female, or nonbinary), they can develop gender dysphoria. Gender dysphoria is experienced in various ways, including as a desire to get rid of one's physical sex characteristics and to have the physical characteristics of the other gender, a desire to be treated as an alternative gender, and a conviction that one's feelings and reactions are more like that of the other gender rather than like those of their assigned sex. The diagnostic criteria for gender dysphoria are included in the American Psychiatric Association's *Diagnostic and Statistical Manual of Mental Disorders* (*DSM–5*), but gender dysphoria is not a mental illness. Nevertheless, the mismatch between assigned sex and the internal perception of being a different gender can cause severe distress that may result in other mental health problems. Gender dysphoria is different from nonconforming sexual orientation (see question 26).

People experiencing gender dysphoria may take steps to make the way they present themselves to the world and the way the world sees them consistent with their own perception of their gender identity as a way to reduce stress and improve their psychological and social functioning. Some nonhormonal steps can include changing one's name and pronouns, changing one's gender on official documents, and changing one's style of dress.

Many people experiencing stressful gender dysphoria also seek medical help to transition to a different gender. Physicians require a full physical workup and usually a behavioral health evaluation before they will proceed with transition therapy. Hormone therapy carries specific risks and may not be suitable for people who have certain medical conditions such as hormone-sensitive cancers or a history of blood clots (deep vein thrombosis). It is important for the transitioning individual to understand the risks involved in treatment and to be able to give informed consent to the treatment plan. Transitioning individuals who work with a mental health professional in addition to a doctor specializing in transition medicine are more likely to be satisfied with the results of treatment.

Feminizing hormone therapy is given to males who want to transition to females. This therapy helps align their body with their gender identity. During feminizing hormone therapy, the individual takes medication to block the production of testosterone by their male organs. They will also take estrogen to promote the formation of female secondary sex characteristics (see case illustration 2). Taking these drugs will result in decreased sex drive; decreased erections; shrinkage of the testes, resulting in infertility; breast development; less oily skin; decreased facial hair; redistribution of body fat; and decreased muscle mass. The process is gradual and can take two to three years to complete.

Masculinizing hormone therapy is given to females who want to transition to males in order to align their body with their gender identity.

During masculinizing hormone therapy, the individual takes gradually increasing doses of testosterone by injection or through a skin gel. This stops menstruation, resulting in infertility. It also causes the voice to deepen, increases the growth of facial and body hair, increases muscle mass and strength, and causes body fat to be redistributed. Some individuals also participate in voice therapy to lower the voice and make it sound more masculine.

After hormone therapy, some individuals seek gender affirmation surgery (formerly called sex reassignment surgery) that will give them physical organs that match their gender identity. Common surgeries include facial surgery to make features more masculine or feminine, surgery to increase or reduce breast size, and surgery to transform or reconstruct genital organs. As of 2020, about 0.6% of people in the United States identified as transgender.

Hormones Regulating Basic Body Functions

28. What body functions does the thyroid affect?

The thyroid gland is a small bat-shaped piece of tissue located in the neck in front of the Adam's apple with a "wing" of the bat on either side of the windpipe (trachea). In adults the gland weighs between 1 and 2 oz (30–60 g) and measures about 2 in (5 cm) across. Despite its small size, the thyroid influences most critical body functions, including heart rate, breathing rate, body temperature, rate of digestion, body weight, menstrual cycles, sperm maturation, muscle strength, cholesterol level, sleep quality, and in young children, growth and brain maturation. It controls the rate of cellular metabolism by adjusting the amount of oxygen a cell uses and by stimulating cells to produce proteins that regulate these vital body functions.

The thyroid produces the hormones thyroxine (T4) and triiodothyronine (T3). T4 makes up about 80% of the hormone secreted by the thyroid; however, T3 is the more potent and biologically active hormone. Most T4 is converted to T3 in cells. To make T3 and T4, the thyroid needs to take in iodine that circulates in the blood. Iodine is an essential trace mineral that the body must acquire from outside food sources. Good natural sources of iodine include seaweed (e.g., nori, kelp, kombu), salt water fish (e.g., cod, tuna), and seafood. In the early 1900s, before fish and seafood could safely be transported long distances, iodine deficiency was a major problem in the inland parts of the United States and in landlocked countries. In 1920, salt manufacturers in the United States began voluntarily adding iodine to table salt. This practically eliminated the problem of iodine deficiency. Today about 120 countries require that iodine be added to salt. This has significantly reduced thyroid deficiency disorders (see question 29).

Control of thyroid hormones begins in the hypothalamus, a part of the brain that connects the nervous system to the endocrine system. The hypothalamus secretes thyrotropin-releasing hormone (TRH). A releasing hormone is a protein made in the hypothalamus that causes the anterior pituitary, a nearby endocrine tissue, to make another hormone. In this case, TRH stimulates the anterior pituitary to make and release into the bloodstream thyroid-stimulating hormone (TSH). TSH, in turn, stimulates the thyroid to secrete T3 and T4.

Some actions of thyroid hormone include increasing one's heart rate, increasing the strength of heart contractions, controlling the speed at which nutrients are absorbed from the intestine, and regulating body temperature. Temperature regulation occurs because the presence of increased thyroid hormone in the blood makes the blood vessels relax and become more elastic. This allows more heat to escape the body. When less thyroid hormone is present, the vessels contract, slowing heat loss. The contracting and relaxing of blood vessels also affect blood pressure. Taken together, the actions of thyroid hormones control the metabolic rate, which is the speed at which the body uses energy supplies.

Thyroid hormone production is controlled by an exquisitely sensitive negative feedback loop. Sensors in the hypothalamus monitor the amount of T3 and T4 circulating in the body. When the hypothalamus senses there is too much thyroid hormone in the blood, it stops making TRH. The absence of TRH tells the pituitary to stop making TSH. Without TSH, the thyroid stops making T3 and T4. When T3 and T4 levels become too low, the hypothalamus begins making TRH, and the process of thyroid hormone production begins again.

A third hormone called calcitonin also comes from the thyroid. Calcitonin is produced by specialized C-cells embedded within the thyroid. This hormone helps to regulate calcium levels in the body, and its production is unrelated to T3 and T4 production. When calcium levels in the blood are too high, calcitonin lowers blood calcium by stimulating the incorporation of calcium into bone and increasing the amount of calcium excreted in urine. Calcitonin production is not affected by the TRH-TSH-thyroid hormone loop. For more on calcitonin, see question 9.

29. What happens if my thyroid over- or underproduces thyroid hormones?

Thyroid hormones help regulate most basic body functions, so an underactive thyroid (hypothyroidism) or an overactive thyroid (hyperthyroidism) affects general health and well-being. An estimated 1 in 20 Americans has abnormal thyroid hormone values, although many people are unaware of this and remain undiagnosed because they show few symptoms. People of all ages and races can develop thyroid disorders, but they are most common in women, people over age 60, and those with type 1 or type 2 diabetes (see question 35) or an autoimmune disease.

Blood tests are used to check for thyroid functioning. The first test usually measures thyroid-stimulating hormone (TSH; see question 28). High levels of TSH indicate that the thyroid is not adequately responding to stimulation and is producing too little thyroid hormone. Blood tests can also measure the amount of the hormones thyroxine (T4) and triiodothyronine (T3).

Hypothyroidism is much more common than hyperthyroidism. Hypothyroidism slows the body's metabolism. Symptoms of hypothyroidism are general and often overlooked or attributed to other conditions. These can include fatigue, difficulty concentrating, trouble sleeping, depression, unusual sensitivity to cold, dry skin, brittle nails, joint and muscle pain, unexplained weight gain, heavy and prolonged menstrual bleeding, and sometimes, difficulty becoming pregnant. Hypothyroidism is successfully treated with levothyroxine (Levoxyl, Synthroid, Tirosint), a thyroid hormone replacement pill that is taken daily.

Iodine deficiency is the most common cause of hypothyroidism worldwide. The body must acquire iodine from outside food sources to make thyroid hormones. After surveying data from 130 countries, the World Health Organization determined that about 30% of the world's population is iodine deficient. Iodine-deficient people have difficulty making enough thyroid hormone. They often develop an enlarged thyroid that causes a swelling in the neck called a goiter. Goiters can also be caused by immune system disorders that affect the thyroid.

Hashimoto thyroiditis is the most common cause of hypothyroidism in the United States. Thyroiditis is inflammation of the thyroid. Hashimoto thyroiditis is an autoimmune disorder in which the body's immune system inappropriately attacks healthy thyroid cells, causing inflammation and decreased function. Hashimoto thyroiditis tends to run in families. Another type of thyroiditis called postpartum thyroiditis causes hypothyroidism in 5%–9% of women after childbirth. The condition is almost always temporary, and even without treatment, thyroid hormone levels rise to normal after a few months.

Hypothyroidism can also affect newborns. The thyroid gland is the first gland to form in the fetus. It begins to develop around week five of pregnancy. About 1 in 4,000 babies is born with a thyroid gland that failed to develop properly. Left untreated, these babies develop serious mental and physical disabilities. In most states, a newborn blood test checks for thyroid hormone levels. Once identified, lifelong thyroid hormone replacement allows these babies to develop normally.

Hyperthyroidism speeds up the body's metabolism. Symptoms of an overactive thyroid can include rapid or irregular heartbeat, nervousness, anxiety, irritability, increased sweating, excessive sensitivity to heat, trouble sleeping, fatigue, light or irregular menstrual periods, muscle and joint aches, frequent bowel movements, unintentional weight loss, trembling hands, and goiter.

Graves' disease is the cause of on an overactive thyroid in more than 70% of people who have hyperthyroidism. This disease is caused by the immune system producing antibodies (the proteins that normally fight foreign invaders such as bacteria) that inappropriately stimulate the thyroid to overproduce thyroid hormone. Graves' disease causes a symptom called Graves' ophthalmopathy that is not found in other causes of hyperthyroidism. This symptom causes the eyes to become inflamed. The tissue around the eyes then swells, making the eyes bulge.

Hyperthyroidism can be treated with medications that interfere with the production of thyroid hormone. In the United States, this is generally the preferred treatment. Some people react badly to antithyroid medication. An alternative is the injection of radioactive iodine into the thyroid to damage the cells that make thyroid hormones. Surgery to remove all or part of the thyroid is also an option. If the entire thyroid is removed, thyroid hormone replacement medication must be taken. The choice of treatment depends on the individual's age, health status, and the cause of the hyperthyroidism.

30. How do hormones regulate fluid balance in your body?

You come in from a run hot, sweaty, and thirsty, so you chug down a glass of water. Almost instantly, long before the water you drink gets absorbed into your bloodstream, the sensation of thirst disappears. So how does the body sense that you need water and then immediately sense when you have had enough?

Water is essential to life. People can live longer without food than without water. Most water is acquired through food and drink and is absorbed through the digestive system, although a small amount is a byproduct of the metabolic activity of cells in the body. The body of a 154 lb (70 kg) man contains around 10.5 gal (42 L) of water. About 92% of this water is found in or surrounding cells, but it is the 8% in blood that is affected by hormones that maintain fluid balance.

In addition to water, blood contains electrolytes. These are inorganic compounds that dissolve in water to form charged ions. Salt (NaCl), for example, breaks down into Na^+ and Cl^-. The ratio of dissolved electrolytes to fluid is called osmolarity. Blood osmolarity must stay within a very narrow range for the body to function properly. Na^+ and potassium (K^+) are the two main electrolytes that determine blood osmolarity. Their concentration in blood is regulated by the action of two hormones on the kidneys.

Some small amount of water is lost through perspiration and in air exhaled from the lungs, but most leaves the body as urine produced by the kidneys. Each kidney contains about two million filtering units called nephrons. Each nephron consists of a knot of tiny blood vessels called the glomerulus and a tubule. As blood flows into the glomerulus, water, ions such as Na^+, and small molecules are filtered out of the blood and into the tubule. Antidiuretic hormone (ADH, also known as vasopressin) and aldosterone act on the tubules to determine how many ions (mostly Na^+ and K^+) and how much water is reabsorbed into the bloodstream and how much is excreted as urine to maintain fluid balance in the body.

ADH is a hormone made in the hypothalamus. Special osmoreceptors that respond to changes in fluid balance are located in the hypothalamus. They continuously monitor the osmolarity of blood. When the osmolarity of blood increases (i.e., when the ratio of ions to fluid increases), the hypothalamus is triggered to produce ADH. ADH is transported to the nearby posterior pituitary, from which it is released into the bloodstream. It interacts with the tubules in the nephrons in a way that allows more water to be reabsorbed from the tubules. The result is that water is conserved in the body, and a smaller amount of concentrated urine is excreted. When a person drinks a large amount of liquid, ADH production is inhibited. Less water moves from the nephron tubules back into the blood, and a large amount of dilute urine is produced. (See question 40 for how drinking alcohol affects this process.)

The hormone aldosterone also acts on the kidneys to maintain blood homeostasis. It is part of a complex system of proteins and enzymes called the renin-angiotensin-aldosterone system that mainly regulates blood pressure. Aldosterone is made by the adrenal cortex. Its production is triggered by decreasing blood levels of Na^+, increasing levels of K^+, low blood volume, and/or low blood pressure. Aldosterone acts on kidney tubules so that they reabsorb more Na^+. This also increases the reabsorption of water to balance the increased amount of Na^+ entering the blood. At the same time, aldosterone increases the amount of K^+ excreted in urine.

Osmoreceptors in the hypothalamus monitor blood osmolarity. In the long term, they do an excellent job of maintaining fluid balance, but one question remains. If it takes at least 10 minutes for the water you drink to be absorbed from the digestive system and for the change in osmolarity to be detected by the hypothalamus, why don't you keep on gulping down water for 10 minutes after your exercise? Why does the sensation of thirst stop almost immediately after you drink something?

Most research on this question has been done on laboratory animals, but a similar mechanism appears to work in humans. A specialized part of the brain called the lamina terminalis appears to play a major role in controlling the sensation of thirst. Stimulating neurons in this part of the brain has been shown to stimulate thirst and drinking behavior in animals. However, when scientists looked at these neurons over time, they found that their activity decreased with each swallow of a liquid. As a result, the sensation of thirst and desire to drink was turned off long before any of the liquid consumed could be absorbed into the bloodstream and detected by the osmoreceptors in the hypothalamus.

31. How does the body respond to fear and stress?

As you drive down a busy street, a bicyclist pedals through a stop sign and crosses in front of your car. You slam on the brakes and miss the cyclist. Epinephrine has saved you from having an accident. But now that the danger has passed, your hands are shaking, your heart is pounding, and you are breathing fast. You need to pull over and wait for a few minutes before you feel comfortable driving on.

Short-term stress

Epinephrine (also called adrenaline) is known as the "fight or flight" hormone. It is produced by the adrenal medulla. The adrenal glands, located above each kidney, are small triangular organs that measure about 1.5×3 in (3.8×7.6 cm). They consist of two layers that produce different hormones with different functions. The outer layer, called the adrenal cortex, produces hydrocortisone, commonly called cortisol, and aldosterone, a hormone involved in fluid balance (see question 30). The inner layer, called the adrenal medulla, produces epinephrine and norepinephrine (also called noradrenaline).

Epinephrine is secreted by modified nerve cells in the adrenal medulla. When you sense danger, a message is sent through the nervous system to the hypothalamus in the brain. The hypothalamus then notifies the adrenal medulla by way of nerve impulses to release epinephrine. This response is completely involuntary and happens within a fraction of a second.

Epinephrine prepares the body for fight or flight. Heart rate increases, and blood is temporarily shifted away from less essential functions such as digestion and excretion and is increased in the brain and muscles so that they are ready for action. The small airways of the lungs dilate to make more oxygen available. Glucose stored in the liver is released into the bloodstream for increased energy. Sensitivity to pain is decreased, which is why people can continue to run or fight when injured. The response to epinephrine is short lived. Once the threat is over, the individual is left panting, with a pounding heart, dry mouth, and shakiness or dizziness. It takes much more time for the body to calm down and return to normal than it does to gear up for action.

People who experience post-traumatic stress syndrome (PTSD) often have inappropriate epinephrine surges in response to perceived or imagined dangers. For example, a car backfire may trigger PTSD and an epinephrine response in a combat veteran. Some people even have these surges in response to triggering mental images or memories. Other people actually enjoy the feeling of the epinephrine rush that they get during activities such as skydiving, riding a roller coaster, bungee jumping, or watching a horror movie.

Epinephrine is also used as a drug to treat anaphylaxis. Anaphylaxis is a severe, potentially fatal, allergic reaction that sends the body into shock. People who are allergic to bee stings or a common food such as peanuts often carry a pen-like device that allows them to inject themselves with a premeasured amount of epinephrine if they are exposed to a substance that triggers their allergy. This injection helps to counteract the effects brought on by the allergic reaction.

A second hormone, norepinephrine, is also secreted by the adrenal medulla in response to fear and sudden stress. It is produced in much smaller quantities than epinephrine. Norepinephrine is both a hormone and a neurotransmitter. Most norepinephrine is secreted in nonemergency situations by nerve endings, but in a threatening situation, it is also secreted by the adrenal medulla. Norepinephrine plays a role in mood and the ability to concentrate. In high-stress situations, it helps to increase focus, prepares the body for exercise, and acts as a supplement to epinephrine.

Long-term stress

Not all stress is immediate and short lived. Illness, injury, family conflict, financial or job worries, and relationship concerns can cause less obvious but long-term stress. Cortisol, secreted by the adrenal cortex, is often called the stress hormone. To some degree, this is unfair. Cortisol plays a role in regulating many essential body functions, including metabolism, blood glucose levels, salt and water balance, and blood pressure. It also helps to reduce inflammation, improves alertness, and affects the formation of memories. In pregnant women, cortisol is needed for proper development of the fetus. Nevertheless, when a person experiences prolonged stress, the resulting high levels of cortisol can damage health.

The production of cortisol is controlled by the hypothalamus, which secretes corticotropin-releasing hormone (CRH). CRH signals the anterior pituitary to produce adrenocorticotropic hormone (ACTH). ACTH travels through the bloodstream and stimulates the adrenal cortex to secrete cortisol. Aldosterone, which plays a role in fluid balance, is also produced by the adrenal cortex, but it is activated by a different system.

Long-term exposure to high levels of cortisol can result in high levels of blood glucose, increased blood pressure, decreased thyroid function (see question 28), acne, slow wound healing, easy bruising, increased susceptibility to disease, decreased muscle strength, weight gain, and major fatigue. Long-term overexposure to cortisol has also been implicated in anxiety, depression, sleep problems, and problems concentrating or "brain fog."

Diseases of the adrenal glands are uncommon. Cushing's syndrome is a disorder where the adrenal cortex produces too much cortisol. This disease affects only between 40 and 70 people per million. It can be caused by a tumor of the pituitary gland or of the adrenal. Addison's disease is the opposite of Cushing's syndrome and is also rare. People with Addison's disease do not produce enough adrenal cortex hormones. Former president John F. Kennedy is probably the most famous person to be treated for Addison's disease. He kept his diagnosis secret for political reasons, and those around him claimed his health issues had other causes.

32. Why do teens find it hard to fall asleep early?

Parents often complain that their teens stay up too late and do not get enough sleep. According to the Sleep Foundation, adolescents need between 8 and 9 hours of sleep each night, but because they tend to go to bed late and get up early for school, they average only between 6.5 and 7 hours. Teens counter that they stay up because they do not feel sleepy much before 11:00 p.m. And they are correct. Timing of the secretion of the hormone melatonin changes at puberty, pushing adolescents naturally toward a later bedtime.

Melatonin is produced in the pineal gland, a tiny triangular gland located deep in the brain and weighing only 0.0004 oz (0.1 g). This hormone was not isolated until 1958, when Aaron Lerner and colleagues at Yale University discovered melatonin while working on a project involving frogs. Most vertebrates have a pineal gland, and all living things—bacteria, fungi, plants, and animals—produce melatonin. Many cells in the body, including those in the ovary, blood vessels, and intestine have receptors for melatonin, but melatonin's function in relation to these organs is not well understood.

Melatonin plays a role in the regulation of circadian rhythms, the natural internal 24-hour clock found in all living things. In humans, secretion of the hormone influences the sleep-wake cycle. When light hits photoreceptors in the eye, nerves signal the hypothalamus. Neurons from the hypothalamus then signal the pineal gland to prevent it from secreting melatonin. As it grows dark, less light enters the eye. Signals to the hypothalamus slow, so the hypothalamus stops sending inhibiting signals to the pineal. Without the inhibiting signals, the pineal begins secreting melatonin. Melatonin does not actually put a person to sleep. Instead, it prepares the body for sleep by slightly lowering body temperature, slowing breathing, lowering blood pressure, and producing feelings of tiredness.

For reasons scientists do not understand, at puberty melatonin naturally shifts to being secreted later in the evening. As a result, melatonin-moderated feelings of tiredness begin about two hours later in many healthy adolescents. The shift often moves sleepiness from around 9:00 p.m. to about 11:00 p.m. In extreme cases, a condition develops called delayed sleep phase disorder, in which the person simply cannot fall asleep until late at night. Although delayed sleep phase disorder affects only 1 or 2 of every 100 adults, the Sleep Foundation has found that it affects about 16 of every 100 teenagers.

Of course, there are nonhormonal reasons teenagers stay up late such as finishing homework, chatting on social media, or becoming engrossed in a book, television show, or video game. Research has shown that the wavelength of light from screens—computers, iPads, and smartphones—is especially stimulating to the hypothalamus and good at preventing the secretion of melatonin. To make falling asleep easier, the Sleep Foundation recommends spending some time outdoors in natural sunlight every day, turning off screens one hour before going to bed, and maintaining a regular sleep-wake schedule.

Synthetic melatonin is sold as a dietary supplement intended to be used as a sleep aid. In the United States and Canada, it is sold over the counter. In the European Union and Australia, it can only be purchased by prescription. One well-controlled study found that people who took melatonin about an hour before bedtime fell asleep seven minutes faster than those who did not. Other studies have found that melatonin can help overcome jet lag, but only if it is taken at the proper time and other adjustments such as avoiding caffeine are made. Claims have been made that supplemental melatonin helps shift workers adjust to shift work, promotes eye health, treats stomach ulcers and heartburn, and increases growth hormone in men. These claims have not been substantiated in rigorous, unbiased clinical trials.

General medical opinion suggests that supplemental melatonin taken at a low dose for a short time may help with sleep difficulties, but that one should consult a doctor first. Even though low doses of supplemental melatonin appear to have few side effects, some people, including pregnant and breastfeeding women, and people with depression, an autoimmune disorder, or a seizure disorder should not use it.

Another thing to consider if planning to take melatonin as a sleep aid is that as a dietary supplement, melatonin is not regulated or approved by the FDA. A 2017 study by the American Academy of Sleep Medicine found that the amount of melatonin in 71% of the samples tested was more than 10% or less than 10% of the amount listed on the label. The actual amounts ranged from 83% less to 478% more than the labeled amount, another reason to seek a doctor's advice before using this supplement.

33. How do your hormone levels change as you get older?

Everyone's body changes as they grow older. Growth hormone makes children grow taller (see question 7). At puberty, sex hormones remodel the body of boys into men (see question 23) and that of girls into women (see question 13). These changes are universal and involuntary because they are driven by the innate interplay between hormones and the body's metabolic processes.

In adulthood, changes to the body become more subtle. Adults do not keep growing taller. Intentional exercise and dietary choices may change the shape of adult bodies, but except during pregnancy (see question 20), these changes are not preprogramed by hormones. Nevertheless, with increasing age, the levels of many hormones and their effects on target tissues change. At first, these changes are imperceptible. Later, many can be detected by blood tests, and eventually, the changes are reflected in the in physical and behavioral changes associated with old age.

Researchers do not completely understand the biochemical mechanisms that control the aging process, but they do know that changes in hormone levels and the body's metabolic rate are involved. As people age, the hypothalamus continues to secrete about the same amount of releasing hormones (see question 2). The anterior pituitary, which responds to releasing hormones by secreting other hormones, reaches its greatest size in middle age. After that, it begins to shrink and becomes less responsive to hormones from the hypothalamus. This results in a decrease in anterior pituitary hormones. The second thing that occurs during aging is that the target tissues of certain hormones become less sensitive to the hormone and respond less strongly. This is often true, for example, of the cellular response to insulin (see question 34).

The clearest example of hormone-driven change due to aging occurs in women when they enter menopause. Menopause, or the end of menstrual periods and fertility, can normally begin any time between ages 40 and 55. The process occurs gradually in all women, and for a time known as perimenopause ("around menopause"), the levels of hormones fluctuate widely, giving rise to symptoms such as hot flashes, night sweats, emotional ups and downs, and irregular menstrual periods. Ultimately, the anterior pituitary no longer secretes enough luteinizing hormone (LH) and follicle-stimulating hormone (FSH) to cause an egg to mature and the ovary to produce the estrogen spike that releases an egg (see question 15). With no egg, conception is not possible, and menstrual bleeding stops.

Some experts in male health believe that men undergo a similar period called male menopause or, more technically, andropause. Male menopause is not a proven condition, and its existence is debatable. Testosterone levels in men peak around age 20. After age 30, they begin to decline by about 1% each year. Initially, this decline has no effect on sex drive or sexual performance.

Around age 50, some men begin to experience low energy, depression, reduced muscle mass, increased body fat, reduced sex drive, and sometimes problems maintaining erections. Some doctors define this collection of symptoms as male menopause. Others do not because unlike menopause in women, not all men experience these symptoms, and the male reproductive system does not completely shut down as it does for women. Men still make sperm and, unless incapable of having an erection, can still father children well into old age. Male menopause symptoms rarely are reversed by taking supplemental testosterone, a treatment that can have serious side effects. Since many symptoms of male menopause can be caused by other conditions such as type 2 diabetes or circulatory problems, the verdict on whether male menopause is a specific syndrome remains open.

Other hormonal changes with aging are less obvious. The thyroid tends to produce less thyroid hormone. This slows the metabolic rate of cells, which in turn causes the body to produce less heat, explaining why the elderly often feel cold. Parathyroid hormone, which controls calcium levels in the blood (see question 11) increases. This means more calcium is dissolved out of bones, resulting in weaker, more easily broken bones in the elderly.

As people age, blood glucose levels spike more rapidly after meals and often stabilize at higher-than-normal values, causing type 2 diabetes. This occurs because the target cells become less sensitive to insulin, the hormone that controls blood glucose levels and/or less insulin is produced (see question 34). The pineal gland becomes calcified and produces less melatonin as people age, which suggests a reason why the elderly often have difficulty with sleep-wake cycles. Aldosterone production by the adrenal cortex decreases. This can cause a drop in blood pressure and a decrease in the sensation of thirst. Although the production of many hormones changes with age, cortisol, epinephrine, and norepinephrine remain at fairly constant levels throughout life.

·❖·

Hormones Regulating Nutrients and Appetite

34. How is blood glucose regulated, and why does it matter?

All cells use glucose for energy. Glucose is a simple sugar made of carbon, hydrogen, and oxygen. In the body it comes from the breakdown of complex carbohydrates in starchy foods such as pasta, potatoes, rice, and bread and as naturally occurring sugar in fruits. These sources normally provide all the glucose the body needs. Humans have a strong preference for foods that taste sweet. In industrialized societies, sugar or corn syrup is often added by manufacturers to processed foods, cake, cookies, candy, and soft drinks or added by individuals to coffee or tea to make these foods taste more appealing.

The American Heart Association (AHA) recommends that for health reasons, women should consume no more than 6 tsp (24 g) or 100 calories of added sugar and men no more than 9 tsp (36 g) or 150 calories daily. For reference, one 12 oz can of Coke contains almost 10 tsp (39 g) of added sugar. According the Harvard University School of Public Health, Americans far exceed the AHA recommendation, consuming an average of 22 tsp (88 g) of added sugar, or an extra 350 calories, daily. Over time, this added sugar can overwhelm hormonal mechanisms that keep blood glucose levels within healthy limits.

The major regulators of blood glucose are hormones made in the pancreas. The pancreas is a small organ about 6 in (15 cm) long and weighing about 3 oz (85 g). It is located behind the stomach on the upper left side of the body. About 95% of cells in the pancreas are exocrine cells. They secrete a mixture of water and digestive enzymes into a duct that carries the fluid to the small intestine where it aids in digestion. The other 5% of pancreatic cells are endocrine cells that exist in clumps called islets scattered throughout the pancreas. They secrete hormones directly into the bloodstream. Two main types of islet cells produce the hormones that regulate glucose levels. In a healthy person, these hormones act in opposition to each other to keep the amount of glucose in the blood within narrow, healthy limits.

When blood glucose levels begin to rise, for example after eating a meal, beta cells in the pancreas are triggered to secrete the hormone insulin. This hormone does four things to help reduce the level of glucose in the blood.

- Insulin allows glucose to enter cells. All cells have receptors for insulin embedded in their membranes. When a molecule of insulin meets a cellular receptor, it binds to the receptor in a way that opens a channel that allows glucose to leave the bloodstream and enter the cell where it is used for energy.
- Insulin acts on the liver so that it takes in glucose and converts it into glycogen. Glycogen is basically a series of linked glucose molecules that have been removed from the blood and stored in the liver until they are needed for energy.
- Insulin acts on skeletal muscles to increase their uptake of glucose. Skeletal muscles also convert glucose to glycogen. The difference between skeletal muscles and the liver is that glycogen in skeletal muscles can be broken down into glucose, but it can only be used by those muscles, for example, during exercise. Glycogen stored in the liver can be released into the bloodstream and used anywhere in the body.
- Insulin signals the hypothalamus in the brain to suppress feelings of hunger so that the individual stops eating.

About four to six hours after eating a meal or sooner after exercise, blood glucose levels drop below the normal set point. This causes alpha cells in the pancreas to secrete the hormone glucagon. Glucagon signals the liver to break down glycogen into glucose and release it into the bloodstream. Beta cells, in addition to producing insulin, also produce a hormone called amylin. This hormone was not discovered until 1987. It acts as a brake on glucagon production to keep blood glucose levels from getting too high. It also slows digestion and the absorption of glucose from the small intestine.

Blood glucose levels are measured with simple blood tests. A fasting glucose test measures the amount of glucose in the blood after eating no food for at least eight hours. A healthy value is less than 100 mg/dL (5.6 mmol/L). An oral glucose test measures glucose in the blood two hours after drinking a sugary liquid. A healthy value is 140 mg/dL (7.8 mmol/L). When a person's blood glucose measures between 100 mg/dL and 125 mg/dL (6.5–7.0 mmol/L), the individual is diagnosed with prediabetes. Exercise and changes in diet can often reduce prediabetes glucose levels to healthy levels. When glucose values are 126 mg/dL (7.0 mmol/L) or higher, the individual has diabetes and needs medical intervention.

The glycosylated hemoglobin test (A1c) is a test that measures the average glucose in the blood over the preceding three months. Glucose binds with hemoglobin, the molecule in red blood cells that carries oxygen throughout the body. The amount of bound hemoglobin can be measured. The higher the amount of glucose in the blood, the greater the amount bound to hemoglobin. The life span of a red blood cell is about three months, so A1c measures a moving three-month average of the percentage of glucose bound to hemoglobin. A healthy A1c value is less than 5.7%. Prediabetes values are from 5.7% to 6.4%. Anything higher indicates diabetes.

35. How do type 1 and type 2 diabetes differ?

Diabetes is a metabolic disorder caused by consistently high levels of glucose in the blood. It is not contagious. The two most common types of diabetes are called type 1 and type 2 diabetes. They develop because of failures at different points in the glucose regulation system (see question 34). This means the risk factors for developing each type of diabetes are different, and each type has a somewhat different treatment. Regardless of the type of diabetes, uncontrolled high levels of glucose can damage blood vessels, increase the risk of heart attack and stroke, cause blurry vision or blindness, damage nerves in the feet and legs, make the individual more susceptible to infections, keep wounds from healing, and cause sexual dysfunction in both men and women.

Type 1 diabetes

Type 1 diabetes, formerly called juvenile diabetes, is found in only about 5% of people diagnosed with diabetes. It is a life-threatening autoimmune disorder. In an autoimmune disorder, an error in the body's immune system causes it to attack and destroy normal healthy body cells. Graves' disease (see question 29), celiac disease, and rheumatoid arthritis are other examples of autoimmune disorders. In the case of type 1 diabetes, the immune system attacks and destroys beta cells in the pancreas. This means the body cannot make insulin. Without insulin, glucose cannot enter cells, so it builds up to toxic levels in the blood. Before 1921 when insulin was isolated and purified by a team of four Canadian researchers (see question 3), a diagnosis of type 1 diabetes was a death sentence.

Signs of type 1 diabetes develop suddenly, usually during childhood after about 80% of beta cells have been destroyed. It is unclear why some people develop type 1 diabetes, although researchers think it may arise from a combination of genetic mutations and exposure to certain environmental triggers. An early sign is excessive thirst and excessive urination as the body tries unsuccessfully to take in enough water to balance the increasing concentration of glucose molecules in the blood. Symptoms include extreme fatigue, blurred vision, and a condition called diabetic ketoacidosis (DKA) that is fatal if left untreated. DKA develops because cells cannot get energy from glucose. Instead, the body breaks down fat and muscle for energy. This results in the release of molecules called ketones that make the blood more acidic. When the body can no longer compensate for the extra acidity, the individual will vomit, become weak, go into a coma, and die.

People with type 1 diabetes must receive regular injections of insulin multiple times each day. Originally, all insulin was extracted from pork and beef pancreases that were shipped from slaughterhouses to pharmaceutical manufacturers in refrigerated railroad cars. In 1983, the FDA approved the first synthetic insulin made by the biotechnology company Genentech. Today all insulin in the United States and most countries worldwide is synthetic and comes in many strengths, including low-dose veterinary insulin for cats and dogs and in varieties that are effective for varying periods of time.

In people with type 1 diabetes, the correct dose of insulin varies from person to person and must be calculated day by day and for each meal. Calculating the correct dose involves the individual's current blood glucose reading, the amount of carbohydrates to be eaten, a personal number that correlates to how the individual metabolizes the carbohydrates, and their level of exercise. Insulin cannot be taken by mouth; it is destroyed by stomach acid. Traditionally it has been self-injected by syringe into the abdomen. Today, alternate methods include preloaded insulin pens and insulin pumps attached to the body that provide a continuous supply of insulin with extra doses for meals. The individual must still calculate the correct dosage, and insulin pumps must be programmed by the wearer.

To help determine the correct dosage, diabetics must check their blood glucose level multiple times each day. The most basic way of doing this is by sticking the finger, collecting a drop of blood on a special test strip, and inserting it into a machine that reads the glucose level. Today, technology offers a variety of options. Most insulin pump systems come with a sensor that automatically reads the blood glucose level every five minutes, sends the information to a smartphone, and indicates whether the level is trending up or down. Insulin delivery technology is changing rapidly to provide more convenience and flexibility, but the individual must still take responsibility for calculating the correct dose of insulin based on diet, exercise, and personal factors.

Type 2 diabetes

About 95% of people with diabetes are diagnosed with type 2 diabetes. Most people with type 2 diabetes are overweight or obese, physically inactive, and eat a diet high in added sugar. In the past, type 2 diabetes was almost always diagnosed in people over age 45, but increasingly, children and younger people are developing the disorder. In 2020, 1 in 10 Americans, or 34.2 million people, had type 2 diabetes. Another 88 million people had prediabetes, a condition in which blood glucose levels are higher than normal but not high enough to be diagnosed with diabetes. About 7 in 10 people with prediabetes will progress to diabetes within five years.

People with type 2 diabetes make insulin, but their cells become less responsive to it, a condition called insulin resistance. As resistance increases, cells take in less and less glucose, so blood glucose levels increase. In addition, as type 2 diabetes progresses, most people make less and less insulin, adding to the problem of rising glucose levels. Unlike type 1 diabetes where symptoms develop dramatically, in type 2 diabetes, symptoms develop gradually and are easy to ignore or to ascribe to stress, natural aging, or other causes. By some estimates almost one-third of people who have type 2 diabetes will not know they have the disorder unless they have a blood glucose test. People with prediabetes can often reverse or delay the progression to type 2 diabetes with changes in diet and exercise, but only if they know they have the disorder.

Unlike individuals with type 1 diabetes, people with type 2 diabetes often do not need to use insulin. They may be able to lower their blood glucose level with other medications, dietary restrictions, and increased exercise. There are multiple classes of drugs used to treat type 2 diabetes. Some of these drugs increase the sensitivity of cells to insulin the body makes. Others stimulate beta cells to produce more insulin, while some slow glycogen breakdown in the liver and/or reduce the amount of glucose that is absorbed from the intestine. People with type 2 diabetes need to check their blood glucose levels regularly, but not as often as people with type 1 diabetes who may need to check their levels sometimes as often as seven or eight times each day. Type 2 diabetics also do not have to calculate medication dosages on a daily basis.

Because symptoms develop gradually and are not immediately life threatening, people with type 2 diabetes tend to see the disorder as less serious than it actually is. Long-term complications are the same as for type 1 diabetes. Loss of vision is common, and poor wound healing and foot infections can lead to amputation of the foot or leg.

36. What is the "hunger hormone"?

You had a satisfying lunch four hours ago, and already those hunger pangs in anticipation of dinner have started. Blame it on the "hunger hormone," ghrelin. Ghrelin is a hormone involved in a complex series of metabolic processes that appear to help regulate growth and maintain a stable body weight. The hormone is produced primarily in the stomach, although the small intestine, pancreas, gonads, and adrenal cortex also produce small amounts.

Ghrelin was identified and isolated in 1999 because of its interaction with growth hormone, not because of its appetite-stimulating qualities. Later, it was thought to directly control appetite, but recent research suggests that it plays a more complex role. In addition to stimulating appetite, it promotes the release of growth hormone and interacts with insulin, the hormone that controls blood glucose levels. In this way, ghrelin helps to regulate the body's metabolic rate, energy balance, and long-term body weight stability. Ghrelin may play a role in making it difficult to maintain any weight loss over months and years.

Ghrelin is a short-acting hormone. Its secretion is cyclical. It increases rapidly four to six hours after eating or when dieting or fasting. Once released, ghrelin travels through the bloodstream to the part of the hypothalamus that controls appetite. The hypothalamus then triggers sensations of hunger. Ghrelin is also thought to interact with neurons in the reward center of the brain, which may help explain why people find eating so pleasurable and comforting. Eating decreases the secretion of ghrelin. Foods high in carbohydrates and protein slow the production and release of ghrelin faster than foods high in fats. Conversely, dieting and restricting food intake increases ghrelin secretion.

In addition to pre-mealtime release, ghrelin is also secreted in a 24-hour cycle, rising at night and decreasing during the day. It has been suggested that ghrelin, along with the hormone leptin (see question 37) may play a role in the sleep-wake cycle. Some studies have found that ghrelin secretion increases when people regularly get less than seven hours of sleep each night and that these short-sleep individuals also show an increase in body mass index (BMI). The results are suggestive of a relationship between ghrelin, sleep, and weight gain but are not proven.

Does too much ghrelin cause obesity? Research suggests that the relationship between ghrelin and obesity is not that simple. Studies have found that overweight and obese people actually have less ghrelin compared to healthy-weight people. This suggests that obese people, rather than making more ghrelin, are simply more sensitive to the hormone than lean people. On the other hand, very underweight people with eating disorders such as anorexia nervosa or those who suffer from body wasting due to severe chronic illness develop high levels of ghrelin. This may be the body's last-ditch effort to maintain energy balance when it perceives that it is being starved.

Does too little ghrelin promote weight loss? Again, the answer is unclear. People who have gastric bypass surgery for weight loss tend to have lower levels of ghrelin than people who lose weight by diet and exercise. However, this may be because gastric bypass surgery reduces the size of the stomach. Since most ghrelin is produced in the stomach, it may be that reducing stomach size simply reduces the number of cells that make ghrelin.

Could a weight loss pill that blocks ghrelin secretion be created? Although pharmaceutical companies and dieters would be delighted with such a pill, all attempts at synthesizing compounds that block the action of ghrelin and act as an appetite suppressant and diet aid have so far been unsuccessful, and continuing this line of research does not appear promising.

37. Can a hormone signal that I am full and should stop eating?

Ghrelin is a short-acting hormone that makes you feel hungry (see question 36), but leptin, a hormone that helps to control appetite, works much more slowly and helps regulate body weight and energy metabolism in a more subtle way. Leptin was discovered in 1994 by molecular geneticist Jeffrey Friedman (1954–). Friedman wanted to understand how one recessive mutation could cause mice to lose appetite control and become grossly obese. It turned out that the mutation prevented leptin secretion.

Leptin helps inhibit appetite by decreasing the sensation of hunger. A protein hormone secreted into the bloodstream by fat cells rather than a single endocrine organ, leptin acts on the appetite centers in the hypothalamus. In theory, a person who gains weight by adding fat makes more leptin so that appetite is depressed and the individual eats less. If a person loses weight and loses fat, less leptin is produced so that appetite is stimulated.

Ghrelin is a short-acting hormone that stimulates hunger several times each day. Leptin is a long-acting hormone that changes food intake gradually to maintain body weight and energy homeostasis over the long term. On a short-term basis, other signals from stretch receptors in the stomach signal fullness and the need to stop eating, as do rising blood glucose levels (see question 34). There is some evidence that people have a personal set point for energy stored in fat and that leptin secretion is influenced by genetics.

In a healthy person, leptin works on a negative feedback loop. Consuming too many calories creates more fat cells, resulting in more leptin secretion, less appetite, and a reduction in calories consumed. Consuming too few calories (dieting, fasting, involuntary starvation) results in fat being broken down to meet the energy needs of the body. Less fat means less leptin, resulting in greater appetite and (assuming food is available) more calories consumed. Leptin also affects the reward system in the brain. When leptin levels are low, food looks more appealing, and eating is more pleasurable. When leptin levels are high, food does not seem as appealing, and the pleasure in eating is diminished. If this system worked perfectly, it would mean that every person would effortlessly maintain their genetically determined body weight. But the system can fail.

Leptin resistance is a condition in which the brain fails to respond to leptin. It is similar to insulin resistance discussed in question 34. In obese people leptin secretion is high, so the drive to eat should be suppressed. However, in people with leptin resistance, large amounts of leptin are produced, but the brain does not recognize it and thinks the body is starving. This results in two responses. First, the brain signals that the person should eat more. Second, it lowers the body's metabolic rate so that a leptin-resistant person burns fewer calories when at rest. No wonder it is so hard for many people to lose weight and keep it off.

Leptin resistance is not completely understood, but it is believed to be influenced by inflammation, high levels of fats in the blood, and the individual's personal metabolic set point. Although a healthy diet and exercise will cause weight loss, in people with high leptin resistance, the drive to overeat usually remains. This makes keeping the weight off a constant struggle.

Sometimes leptin is sold over the Internet as a weight loss supplement. These supplements are not approved or regulated by the FDA. Multiple studies have found that many of the supplements do not contain any leptin, and even those that do are ineffective. The only people who are definitively helped by supplemental leptin are those who are born with a rare genetic disorder called Prader-Willi syndrome. These children are a normal weight at birth but have an insatiable appetite and soon become morbidly and life-threateningly obese. Like the mice Jeffrey Friedman studied that had no appetite control and ate their way to obesity, these children cannot make leptin. They are sometimes helped by leptin administered under the supervision of a physician.

How Different Substances
Affect Your Hormones

38. What are endocrine disruptors?

The study of endocrine-disrupting chemicals (EDCs) is relatively new. The term "endocrine disruptor" was developed at a conference in Wisconsin in 1991 to define any chemical or mixture of chemicals that interferes with the normal action of hormones. EDCs were first found in animals when scientists noticed consistent abnormalities in the reproductive systems of various fish and amphibians. So far, over 1,000 manufactured chemicals have been identified as potentially having hormone-disrupting properties. The actual number is probably much larger because only a small percentage of the more than 85,000 synthetically manufactured chemicals have been tested for endocrine-disrupting activity. In addition, a few plants produce natural EDCs.

Most EDCs enter the body through food and drink, although a few are acquired by breathing polluted air or absorbed through the skin during direct contact. In addition, EDCs can pass from mother to child in breast milk. Some EDCs bioaccumulate, meaning they build up in the body rather than being flushed out as waste products.

EDCs are found almost everywhere—in pesticides, many types of plastics, including those used to package and store foods and liquids, industrial lubricants, plastic toys, cleaning products, fragrances, cosmetics, shampoos, and toothpastes. EDCs leach into the water supply from toxic waste sites and enter waterways when manufacturers discharge wastewater into streams or rivers. Virtually everyone who has been tested for EDCs (a complicated and expensive process) has had some of these chemicals in their body.

EDCs exert their effects when present in exceedingly small quantities (parts per billion or parts per trillion), making them difficult to isolate and measure. They disrupt the action of hormones in several ways.

- They can mimic the action of a natural hormone by binding to cellular receptors for that hormone and activating target cells. This ability to activate the target cells may cause a stronger response than the natural hormone does or trigger a response at the wrong time.
- They can prevent a cell from responding to a natural hormone by blocking the cell's hormone receptors so that the natural hormone cannot bind with the receptor to activate the cell.
- They can block or alter the process by which hormones or hormone receptors are made or the pathways by which they communicate.

Scientists generally agree that EDCs affect the reproductive systems of wildlife, but there is less agreement about their effects in humans. One area of agreement is that fetuses and newborns are most vulnerable to the effects of EDCs because they experience rapid cell division and growth. Toddlers are also thought to be vulnerable because they play outside more and tend to explore the world by putting things in their mouths.

Research on the effects of EDCs is complicated by the fact that some of the consequences of EDC exposure do not show up until puberty or later. For example, one of the first EDCs recognized was diethylstilbestrol (DES). DES was a drug legally prescribed to help prevent nausea and miscarriages from the 1940s until it was outlawed in 1971. Although the drug did help women carry their pregnancies to term, researchers discovered 20 years later that it caused vaginal cancer in many of the women's daughters. Another example of the delayed effect of EDCs comes from research that shows early and frequent exposure to lavender oil, a popular essential oil that contains a natural EDC, causes girls to go through puberty early (around age nine) and boys to develop breasts.

There are multiple classes of EDCs, and each class has varying effects, many of which are still under debate by researchers. The most common effects in both animals and humans appear to be on the reproductive system and involve feminization. Some researchers believe that the decrease in men's sperm count over the past 40 years and an increase in breast cancer in women are due to EDC exposure, but other researchers disagree.

Here are listed some of the more common EDCs, the products in which they are found, and the effects researchers believe they may have on humans. Remember, however, that research on their effects is still being questioned, and additional studies are needed, especially on early exposures that may cause problems that do not appear until later in life.

- Phthalates: Used to make plastics more flexible. Found in food packaging, vinyl flooring, adhesives, detergents, lubricating oils, automotive plastics, fragrances, cosmetics, shampoos. They are believed to cause low sperm count, birth defects, and neurobehavioral abnormalities such as attention deficit hyperactivity disorder.
- Bisphenol A. (BPA): Found in food and beverage storage containers, the lining of some cans, and some dental sealants. They are thought to affect the prostate, increase breast cancer risk, increase blood pressure, promote early puberty, and cause neurobehavioral abnormalities. The FDA has declared low levels of BPA safe, but an investigation is ongoing.
- Polybrominated diphenyl ethers (PBDEs): Used as a flame retardant in textiles, furniture, and building materials. They possibly cause cancer and disrupt thyroid hormone and estrogen functions. These chemicals bioaccumulate, which is a cause for concern.
- Polychlorinated biphenyls (PCBs): Used in lubricants and industrial coolants. They possibly increase the likelihood of skin cancer, liver cancer, and brain cancer. They interfere with thyroid hormone and cause developmental delays and menstrual irregularity.
- Plant hormones: Found in lavender and tea tree essential oils. Phytoestrogens similar to natural estrogens are also found in soy products, licorice, citrus fruits, and fennel. They are thought to stimulate early puberty and may worsen certain hormone-sensitive cancers. Their effect is weaker than natural estrogen.

Since 1970, there has been a fivefold or greater increase in plastic manufacturing, which has increased human exposure to EDCs as well as increasing plastic pollution in the oceans. Experts suggest that the best way to decrease exposure to EDCs is to avoid plastic bottles and plastic food packaging, reduce the use of canned food, choose natural cosmetics and fragrance-free products such as laundry detergents and soaps, and pay attention to research that is being done on EDC chemicals.

39. How do anabolic steroid supplements affect your hormones?

Testosterone was first synthesized in Germany in 1935. Since then, chemists have experimented with producing synthetic variations of the hormone. These variations are known as anabolic steroids or, more precisely, anabolic-androgenic steroids. "Anabolic" refers to the ability of the drug to increase protein synthesis, increase bone and muscle mass, and decrease body fat. "Androgenic" indicates their close relationship to the male hormone testosterone.

Anabolic steroids are prescription drugs in the United States, although they are sold without a prescription in some countries such as Mexico. They may legally be prescribed to treat health conditions such as delayed puberty or muscle wasting in cancer or HIV/AIDS patients, but they are best known as drugs used illicitly to enhance athletic performance.

The first known use of anabolic steroids in athletic competition occurred in the 1954 Olympics among Russian weight lifters. The use of anabolic steroids to boost athletic performance peaked in the 1980s. Concerned about unfair competition and negative health effects when these drugs were misused, the U.S. Congress passed the Anabolic Steroids Act of 1990. This Act made anabolic steroids controlled substances and their sale and possession without a prescription punishable by fines and prison terms. Later, the Anabolic Steroids Control Act of 2004 extended the original Act to include anabolic steroid precursor chemicals. This was an attempt to control the development of new laboratory-synthesized "designer" steroids created specifically to be less easily detectable in blood and urine tests.

At one time anabolic steroids were used mainly by competitive athletes. Today these drugs are banned by most sports organizations, including the International Olympic Committee, National Collegiate Athletic Association, Major League Baseball, the National Basketball Association, the National Football League, and the National Hockey League. Positive tests for an anabolic steroid can end the career of an athlete.

Today male bodybuilders and weight lifters in their 20s and 30s and men who have body dysmorphic disorder (BDD) are the main users of illicit anabolic steroids. BDD is a mental health disorder in which people obsess over what they believe are flaws or weaknesses in their body, even though these supposed imperfections are not noticeable to other people. The illegal steroids often are obtained over the Internet from countries where they are sold without a prescription. Some anabolic steroids are injected, while others are taken as pills, and although they do not give the short-term high of many illicit drugs, they are addictive.

Anabolic steroids have major disruptive effects on the male reproductive system. Because their chemical structure closely resembles testosterone, sensors in the body mistake them for the hormone and signal that an excess of testosterone is present in the blood. This triggers the hypothalamus to stop releasing gonadotropin-releasing hormone (GnRH). Without GnRH, the pituitary does not release follicle-stimulating hormone (FSH) and luteinizing hormone (LH), the hormones needed to stimulate production of testosterone and the maturation of sperm. Gradually, the entire male reproductive cycle slows and then shuts down. With long-term use of anabolic steroids, the following things often occur in men:

- Sperm production decreases.
- Sex drive decreases.
- Testicles shrink in size.
- Erections fail to occur or cannot be maintained.
- Infertility develops.
- Hair loss or baldness occurs.
- Breasts enlarge, a condition in men known as gynecomastia.
- Severe acne develops.
- Prostate cancer risk increases.
- Aggressive, sometimes uncontrolled, behavior increases.
- Mood swings become more common, including paranoia and manic behavior.

Women are much less likely to use anabolic steroids because they find their masculinizing effects unacceptable. When they do, acquiring masculine traits is unavoidable.

- Facial and body hair increase.
- The voice deepens.
- Menstrual cycles become irregular or stop.
- Infertility develops.
- Breasts shrink.
- The clitoris swells.
- Acne increases.
- The skin becomes coarser and oilier.
- Sex drive increases.
- Mood swings become more common, including anger, paranoia, and irrational behavior.

Both men and women who use anabolic steroids are also at risk for high blood pressure, high cholesterol levels, increased blood clots, heart attack, fluid retention, liver damage, and kidney failure. Injecting steroids increases the risk of infection. If needles are shared, serious diseases such as HIV, hepatitis B, and hepatitis C can be transmitted. In addition, anabolic steroids cause bones to age faster and stop growing sooner. In 2020, fewer than 2% of high school students used anabolic steroids. However, adolescents who do take these drugs before the growth spurt that accompanies puberty is finished will have stunted height from premature hardening of the long-bone growth plates.

40. How does drinking alcohol affect your hormones?

Hormones play a key role by communicating with the nervous system to maintain homeostasis, or chemical balance, in the body. So how does drinking alcohol change hormone secretion and affect this balance? The answer depends in part on how much and how frequently a person drinks. The National Institute on Alcohol Abuse and Alcoholism defines moderate drinking for adults as two drinks or fewer in a day for men and one drink or fewer in a day for women. Heavy drinking is defined as more than four drinks on any single day or more than fourteen drinks per week for men. For women, it is defined as more than three drinks on any single day or more than seven drinks per week for women.

Blood glucose levels are regulated by two hormones secreted by the pancreas, insulin and glucagon (see question 34). Studies have found that moderate drinking does not change the amount of insulin the pancreas secretes, but it does temporarily make cells more sensitive to insulin so that they take in glucose from the blood more easily. In the short term, this reduces blood glucose levels. At the same time, alcohol slows or prevents the breakdown of glycogen into glucose, a process that normally occurs in the liver when blood glucose levels drop. These combined responses mean that moderate drinking causes a temporary drop in blood glucose levels.

The response is not the same with heavy alcohol use. With heavy long-term drinking, the pancreas gradually secretes less insulin. At the same time, cells become less responsive to the hormone. The combination of less insulin and greater insulin resistance makes blood glucose levels rise. It is not yet clear why this response is opposite of what occurs with moderate drinking.

In heavy drinkers, blood glucose levels tend to stay high rather than returning to normal levels. This often leads to the development of type 2 diabetes. Type 2 diabetes causes multiple serious complications (see question 35), especially if left untreated. Even when treated, alcohol consumption can interfere with the effectiveness of some type 2 diabetes medications.

Alcohol consumption has a strong effect on the production of sex hormones. In women, regular moderate drinking increases estrogen levels and decreases progesterone levels. This is thought to slightly increase the risk of developing breast cancer.

All women make some testosterone, a hormone primarily associated with men but necessary in much smaller amounts for women's health. Heavy alcohol use increases the amount of testosterone a woman makes. This can cause her to develop coarser, oilier skin; more body hair; and acne.

Heavy alcohol consumption also disrupts the hormones that regulate the menstrual cycle (see question 15). Menstrual cycles become irregular. Some women stop ovulating, even if they continue to have light menstrual bleeding. When this occurs, they cannot become pregnant should they want to have a child. If a woman who drinks alcohol does become pregnant, any alcohol use increases the risk of miscarriage and creates the potential for serious birth defects in the fetus.

Alcohol also has negative effects on the male sex hormones. Short-term alcohol consumption can cause a drop in a man's testosterone level within as little as 30 minutes, although in moderate drinkers, this appears to have no permanent effects. Long-term heavy alcohol use, however, can cause major reproductive problems.

Alcohol acts on the hypothalamus to reduce or prevent the release of gonadotropin-releasing hormone (GnRH). Without adequate GnRH, the pituitary produces little or no follicle-stimulating hormone (FSH) and luteinizing hormone (LH). FSH and LH are necessary for testosterone secretion and the production of healthy sperm (see question 22). Ultimately, long-term heavy drinking damages the cells in the testes (Leydig cells) that produce testosterone. Low testosterone can result in low sex drive, failure to have or maintain an erection, and smaller testicles. Alcohol also damages the cells responsible for the maturation of healthy sperm (Sertoli cells). This results in sperm that fail to mature or have defective motility, low sperm counts, and smaller semen volume.

Some effects of alcohol use are reversible, although improvement can take many weeks. Others, such as liver damage, may be permanent.

Boys who begin drinking heavily before or during early puberty may experience delayed puberty. Testosterone replacement therapy will not counteract all the effects of heavy alcohol use on the male reproductive system.

Alcohol also interferes with calcium metabolism and bone health. It inhibits the secretion of parathyroid hormone (PTH). PTH controls the level of calcium in the blood. When the level falls too low, PTH initiates the freeing of calcium from bones to keep the blood level of calcium steady (see questions 9 and 10). Alcohol also decreases the absorption of calcium acquired from diet by altering the actions of vitamin D, a compound necessary for calcium to leave the small intestine and enter the bloodstream. People who drink heavily are statistically more likely to fall and have accidents. With long-term heavy alcohol use, their bones become weaker and break more easily if they fall. This is especially a problem for elderly drinkers whose bones are already weakened due to natural aging processes.

When a person drinks alcohol, cortisol, often called the stress hormone, increases (see question 31). This happens in both moderate and heavy drinkers. It results in an immediate increase in blood pressure and can lead to stress-associated feelings of anxiety and depression. Not only do cortisol levels increase while drinking, they also increase while one is recovering from intoxication. This can initiate the desire to drink more alcohol to relieve unpleasant stressful feelings. This cycle of drinking, beginning to recover from intoxication, and then drinking again to relieve the unpleasant feelings associated with recovery can lead to alcohol use disorder and helps to explain why it can be difficult to break the pattern of alcohol abuse.

41. How does using marijuana affect your hormones?

Since marijuana (*Cannabis sativa*) has only recently been legalized in some places for medical and recreational use, rigorous controlled studies of its effects on the endocrine system are limited. Marijuana studies on human hormones are difficult to compare, and the results range from uncertain to contradictory. For example, researchers have found that the method of consuming the product—by smoking, eating, or vaping—along with the sex of the individual in the study affects the results. They also have found that some endocrine glands respond differently in people who are habitual marijuana users when compared to occasional users. The results also vary depending on whether the researcher used the natural product or an extract of the psychoactive component. All these variables mean that it is difficult to say with a high degree of certainty exactly what effect using marijuana has on the endocrine system in any particular individual. Additional studies are needed to get consistent results.

Marijuana is a natural product that contains more than 100 different compounds. The ones of research interest are tetrahydrocannabinol (THC) and cannabidiol (CBD). THC is the psychoactive ingredient that alters perception and creates a "high." CBD does not produce this effect. Both THC and CBD contain the same number and type of atoms. The arrangement of the atoms determines the presence or absence of psychoactive effects. Marijuana contains about 12% THC. Hemp, the plant from which CBD is extracted, contains less than 0.3% THC. Hemp is legal. The legality of marijuana and THC extract varies from state to state and country to country. People planning to use marijuana should inform themselves about its legal status in their location.

Marijuana interacts with the endocannabinoid system (ECS) in the body. The ECS was discovered in 1990, and researchers are still trying to clarify its role. The system has of two types of receptors. CB_1 receptors are located in the central nervous system (brain and spinal cord) and a few other sites. THC interacts mainly with CB_1 receptors. This interaction is responsible for most of the drug's psychoactive effects. CB_2 receptors are found primarily in immune system tissues and cells. Their function is not well understood.

The body makes some endocannabinoids on its own. These self-made cannabinoids bind with receptors and appear to be involved in maintaining homeostasis or chemical and energy balance in the body by affecting sleep, mood, metabolism, appetite, growth, and fertility. The cannabinoids in marijuana bind strongly with the ECS receptors in the brain. Since the hypothalamus controls many endocrine functions, it is not surprising that using marijuana can affect the regulation and production of various hormones.

Although many of the effects of marijuana use appear to be negative, there is a great deal of interest in its potential medical use. This is especially true of CBD products that are not psychoactive. As of late 2020, the FDA had approved only two medical uses for marijuana products. Epidiolex is a prescription form of CBD approved for treating seizures associated with two rare diseases. Dronabinol (Marinol, Syndros) and nabilone (Cesamet) are prescription synthetic THC products approved for preventing nausea and vomiting associated with chemotherapy.

Here are some of the hormonal changes that studies suggest are caused by marijuana use. Keep in mind, however, that research on marijuana in humans involves complicated variables, not all of which can be controlled. There is no assurance that these findings apply equally to every individual.

- Marijuana is famous for stimulating appetite or giving users the "munchies." It appears that THC, like self-made endocannabinoids, is involved in regulating food intake and energy balance. Small human studies have found that ghrelin, the "hunger hormone" (see question 36) secreted by the stomach, increases after marijuana use. These studies also found that ghrelin increased more when marijuana was eaten rather than smoked. On the other hand, other studies have found that long-term daily use of marijuana increases the body's sensitivity to leptin, the "fullness" hormone (see question 37), and suppresses weight gain.
- Marijuana appears to decrease the insulin spike that occurs after eating something high in sugar (see question 34). People who ate a brownie containing marijuana showed a smaller short-term increase in insulin than people who ate an equivalent brownie without marijuana.
- Regular marijuana use disrupts both male and female reproductive systems because it suppresses the secretion of gonadotropin-releasing hormone (GnRH) from the hypothalamus. This causes men to make fewer sperm and for testosterone levels to decrease. Women's menstrual cycles tend to become irregular with habitual marijuana use.
- In the short term, marijuana increases the release of cortisol, the stress hormone (see question 31), and suppresses immune system function. It also temporarily increases blood pressure and may increase cholesterol levels.
- Regular marijuana use decreases the amount of thyrotropin-releasing hormone (TRH) from the hypothalamus, which in turn decreases the amount of thyroid-stimulating hormone (TSH) from the pituitary. This leads to a decrease in the production of thyroid hormones (see question 28), which can result in weight gain, fatigue, intolerance of cold, decreased sex drive, and depression.
- The THC in marijuana crosses the placenta and impacts a developing fetus. It also appears to suppress the production of growth hormone in children, although little controlled research has been done on this for ethical reasons.
- Overall, long-term regular marijuana use appears to suppress most of the hormones secreted by the hypothalamus that stimulate the pituitary. This, in turn, suppresses the production of pituitary hormones; alters metabolic functions; and affects sleep, fatigue, and mood.

42. How does caffeine affect your hormones?

Caffeine is a naturally occurring stimulant found in coffee beans, tea leaves, kola nuts that are used to flavor soft drinks, and cacao, a component of chocolate. Synthetic caffeine is also added to some soft drinks, energy drinks, and some pain medications such as Excedrin to boost their pain-reliving qualities. Caffeine is considered a drug because in regular users it can create tolerance—that is, it takes larger and larger amounts to produce the same effect. People appear to have a wide range of sensitivity to caffeine, but many people who regularly consume large amounts develop withdrawal symptoms such as headache and anxiety when they stop.

According to the Mayo Clinic, 400 mg of caffeine per day is generally considered a safe amount for healthy adults, but pregnant women and people with high blood pressure or heart conditions should consider limiting consumption. To put the 400 mg amount in perspective, one 12 oz "tall" Starbucks brewed Pikes Peak Roast coffee contains 235 mg of caffeine. An equivalent amount of McDonald's coffee contains between 90 and 109 mg, and the same amount of black tea has about 67 mg. Other 12 oz caffeinated drinks include Coke, 34 mg; Diet Coke, 46 mg; Mountain Dew, 54 mg; Red Bull, 114 mg; Monster Energy, 138 mg; and Rockstar Punched, 180 mg.

Most researchers who study the effects of caffeine give their research subjects measured amounts of synthetic caffeine. Knowing the exact dose and time when caffeine is taken makes it easier for scientists to compare the effects of different doses. However, in the real world, people do not get caffeine all at once in neatly measured doses. They usually acquire it by consuming caffeinated drinks, often in combination with food. This leaves room for a lot of inconsistency. Consider, for example, the difference in caffeine content between the same amount of coffee from Starbucks and McDonald's. To add to the variability, energy drink manufacturers add sugar and other ingredients such as ginseng, taurine (an amino acid found in meat), and milk thistle extract to their drinks. These may also act as stimulants, making it difficult to determine exactly how much the observed hormonal changes are caused specifically by caffeine. Despite these variables, researchers have come to some consistent conclusions.

Cortisol is a stress hormone produced by the adrenal cortex (see question 31). Normally, it is at its highest level in the morning and gradually decreases throughout the day, reaching its lowest level at night. Studies have shown that caffeine appears to mimic some stress conditions that stimulate the release of cortisol. Cortisol causes glucose to be released from the liver and increases blood pressure, heart rate, and alertness. In addition to raising both cortisol and insulin levels, a moderate dose of caffeine has been found to decrease cellular sensitivity to insulin by 15%. This makes it harder for glucose to leave the blood and enter cells where it is used for energy.

Frequent consumption of caffeine may lead to prolonged secretion of cortisol and extended periods of increased blood pressure and higher glucose levels. Since caffeine is often consumed in sugary drinks or in sweetened coffee or tea, this combination of sugar and caffeine may accelerate insulin resistance and increase the risk of developing type 2 diabetes (see question 35).

Depending on when caffeine is consumed, it may also interfere with normal sleep cycles and memory formation. Quality sleep depends partly on low levels of cortisol and high levels of melatonin at night. Poor-quality sleep is often associated with irritability and/or depression and reduced memory formation.

Norepinephrine (also called noradrenaline) secretion is also changed by caffeine consumption. Norepinephrine is produced in the adrenal medulla in response to stress. It is considered both a hormone and a neurotransmitter. Norepinephrine increases alertness; improves mood; shortens reaction time; causes glucose to be released from the liver; and increases heart rate, blood pressure, and blood flow to muscles. This occurs quickly and naturally when the body experiences sudden stress (see question 31). Caffeine also appears to stimulate the release of norepinephrine. In one study, researchers found that people who drank a commercial energy drink under relaxing conditions produced a spike in norepinephrine almost 75% greater than people who drank a liquid that contained the same amount of sugar as the energy drink but none of the stimulant ingredients. Since commercial energy drinks contain multiple stimulants, this does not prove that caffeine caused the norepinephrine increase, but along with other research, it suggests that caffeine plays a role.

Caffeine can also affect reproductive hormones. Caffeine given in a single large dose of 800 mg (more than most people consume in a day) increased testosterone levels in men by 21%. Lower doses produced smaller increases. In women, research results are conflicting. Some studies show that moderate amounts of caffeine increase the level of estrogen in some women and decrease it in others. The reason for this is unclear, although some researchers believe it is somehow linked to differences in ethnicity.

In addition to affecting the endocrine system, caffeine interacts with neurotransmitters such as dopamine and serotonin in the brain. These chemicals regulate, among other things, mood. Given the complexity of caffeine research and its wide-reaching effects on the body, the only general conclusion that can be drawn at this time is that moderate caffeine use probably is harmless in healthy, nonpregnant adults, and excessive use is best avoided. All this suggests that people who regularly drink caffeinated drinks should be aware of how much caffeine they are consuming every day.

43. How does drinking diet soda affect your hormones?

In a healthy person, blood glucose levels are controlled by the balance between insulin and glucagon (see question 34) based on what the individual eats and how much the individual exercises. Almost all regular sodas are sweetened with high fructose corn syrup, a sweetener made from cornstarch. The body treats high fructose corn syrup like sugar because it breaks down into glucose. When a person drinks a regular soda, the pancreas secretes insulin. Insulin allows glucose to leave the bloodstream and enter cells where it is used for energy. Excess glucose is stored as glycogen in the liver and muscles or enters fat cells. But what happens when a person drinks a soda sweetened with an artificial sweetener that contains no calories and no glucose?

Artificial sweeteners are synthetic chemicals that produce the sensation of sweetness in the mouth. The most common artificial sweeteners are sucralose, aspartame, acesulfame potassium (Ace-K), and sorbitol. Artificial sweeteners must be listed in the ingredient panel of foods even though they have no nutritional value.

Most insulin is secreted by the pancreas in response to increasing levels of glucose in the blood, but between 1% and 3% of the total insulin released occurs before food even reaches the stomach. This is called cephalic phase insulin release, and it prepares the digestive system to receive food. The smell, taste, and chewing of food, especially food containing sugar or carbohydrates, stimulates receptors in the tongue and mouth that signal the pancreas to release insulin. Sugar, high fructose corn syrup, and artificial sweeteners all stimulate the same tongue and mouth receptors even though artificially sweetened foods like diet sodas will not increase glucose levels in the blood.

Studies on the metabolic effects of artificial sweeteners are difficult to compare because they are done with different sweeteners and on different populations (e.g., young vs. old, obese vs. normal weight). In 2019, a group of researchers analyzed 56 different reputable human studies on artificial sweeteners. One of the more consistent findings was that artificial sweeteners initially raise insulin levels. For example, in people given sucralose, the level of insulin in the blood was 20% higher than in people who were given water. Other studies have suggested that the unnecessary insulin release stimulated by artificial sweeteners eventually increases insulin intolerance and accelerates the development of type 2 diabetes in at-risk individuals who are older, obese, and physically inactive (see question 35).

Eating sweet foods has conclusively been shown to increase cravings for more sweet foods. Artificial sweeteners may also increase the desire for sweets by interfering with the way the appetite hormones ghrelin and leptin (see questions 36 and 37) interact with the area of the brain that controls hunger and appetite. In some studies, even when eating the same diet, people drinking diet soda gained about two-thirds as much weight as people in the study drinking the same amount of regular soda. To some scientists this suggests that artificial hormones interfere with the gut microbiome and/or make the body less sensitive to leptin, the hormone that signals fullness.

Although there are indications that artificial sweeteners in diet soda and other products do have an effect on the secretion of insulin and possibly on the secretion of hunger hormones and the message they send to the brain, the results across studies are difficult to compare. The only real conclusions that can be drawn at this point are that insulin secretion is affected, diet soda is not a magic key to weight loss or better health, and more research needs to be done.

44. How does playing video games affect your hormones?

Although examining the relationship between video game play and changes in hormone levels is a relatively new area of research, a link has been found between changes in the levels of the stress hormones cortisol and norepinephrine and game play. In addition, researchers have found changes in testosterone levels in multiplayer team games as well as in people watching live sports competitions. These changes may also apply people to watching streaming e-sports.

Cortisol is secreted by the adrenal cortex, or outer layer of the adrenal gland. Norepinephrine is secreted by the adrenal medulla, or inner layer of the same gland. Both hormones are released in response to a perceived threat in order to prepare the body for fight or flight (see question 31). Changes in the levels of these hormones can be detected in saliva. Cortisol is measured directly from saliva samples, while norepinephrine is measured by analyzing the amount of an enzyme that is produced as soon as norepinephrine is secreted. An increase in cortisol and/or norepinephrine indicates increased stress. This stress is also shown physically by an increase in blood pressure, heart rate, and breathing rate and mentally by increased attentiveness and alertness.

Video games can be separated into various genres and subgenres. Researchers have consistently found that different genres of games affect players' hormones differently. In one study, gamers played four single-player games from different genres: puzzle games, runner games, excitement games, and fear games. Puzzle games are games that require concentration, problem solving, and logic. Runner games create stress by imposing a time challenge on the player. Excitement games are games in which the player must fight off threats to win the game. They tend to be violent and move quickly. Fear games are horror games that contain disgusting or gruesome scenes and graphic, brutal fighting, along with psychological stressors such as weird or threatening sounds.

Researchers found that puzzle games are calming. Levels of both cortisol and norepinephrine consistently decreased in gamers who played puzzle games. Levels of cortisol and norepinephrine increased only by a small amount in gamers who played runner games. Excitement games substantially increased both cortisol and norepinephrine. Fear games increased cortisol by about the same amount as excitement games but caused an exceptionally large increase in norepinephrine, something one would expect from a frightening real-world experience.

Other researchers measured changes in testosterone levels in male gamers who competed as a team against another team when playing violent video games, the equivalent of excitement games described above. They found that in the team-against-team competition, men on the winning team had higher levels of testosterone at the end of the game than at the beginning and much higher levels than the losing team. The authors correlated this increase with increased aggression scores. When men competed as individuals against other men on their own team, the rise in testosterone was significantly less when compared to individual competition against someone from the another team. This suggests that social context plays a role in how aggressive gamers are.

Another set of researchers looked at the testosterone level of male sports fans at a World Cup final soccer match. They found that fans of both sides had an increase in testosterone from daily baseline levels before the game. However, at the end of the game, fans of the winning team had much higher testosterone levels than fans of the losing team. Other researchers found that fans of teams in the Rugby World Cup final had increases in testosterone that correlated to the degree of dedication and emotional involvement they had with their team.

Taken together, these studies suggest that watching sports contests in which a male fan is emotionally invested creates a surge of testosterone. Testosterone is involved in aggression, dominance, and competitiveness, but high testosterone also boosts self-esteem. This boost in self-esteem from increased testosterone may help explain the popularity of watching both live sporting contests and e-sport competitions and in playing certain types of video games.

Case Illustrations

1. PETE WORRIES ABOUT HIS HEIGHT

Pete lived and breathed basketball. His dad, George, had been a starter for a top college team and had been good enough to attract the attention of the pros, but not quite good enough to get signed. George dreamed that Pete might someday have the pro career that had passed him by. Pete shared the dream, not just to please his dad, but because he loved the game.

To give Pete a head start, George enrolled him in a basketball training program at age six and spent hours at home teaching him the basics. Pete became a standout player, good enough to get partial scholarship to a private academy known for its strong basketball program.

At the end of seventh grade, all the boys on the basketball team were about the same height, but when eighth grade started, Pete realized many of his teammates had grown several inches over the summer. Not only where they taller, they looked more solid and muscular. A few had even started sprouting facial hair.

Throughout the year, most of Pete's teammates grew taller and began to develop broad shoulders and narrow waists. A few started shaving. Pete worked hard at developing his basketball skills, but he was increasingly aware that boys who were three, four, or even sometimes six inches taller than him had a definite advantage. This worried him, and his worries were reinforced by frequent comments George made about how tall his teammates and opponents were.

"Dad," Pete said one day at the beginning of ninth grade, "How tall were you when you were my age?"

"I don't exactly remember," George said. "But in ninth grade, I was the second tallest kid on the team."

Between ages 11 and 14, Pete had only gained a little over an inch a year, and he was discouraged.

"Do you think I'm ever going to get taller?" Pete asked. "I mean, look at how tall Mac and Dwayne and Darius are. I used to be as tall as all of them."

George tried to reassure Pete that he would eventually catch up to his teammates, but secretly he was worried. By the time he was Pete's age, he was 6 ft 1 in (185 cm). George had seen advertisements on the Internet for growth hormone (GH) and how it could stimulate increased height and muscle mass. Maybe that was what Pete needed. He read various testimonials and decided it would not hurt to get a GH supplement for Pete.

George ordered something called "growth hormone releaser" pills that promised to stimulate the natural production of GH. The releaser was quite expensive, but George thought it was worth trying. Pete took the pills for several months, but he showed no signs of a growth spurt. Frustrated, George made an appointment for Pete to have a complete physical.

The doctor examined Pete and listened to his concerns about his height. Although Pete appeared healthy, the doctor ordered a series of blood tests to check for hormonal or biochemical imbalances. These all came back normal. The doctor tried to reassure Pete that even if his growth spurt started later than most boys, his final height would not be affected, but Pete was still concerned about how his height would affect his basketball potential. He became despondent, and basketball became less fun.

Abruptly, near the end of ninth grade, Pete developed acne and a voracious appetite. By the time school started in September, he had grown 3 in and put on 15 lb (6.8 kg) of mostly muscle. His growth spurt continued, and by the time he graduated from high school, he was a muscular 6 ft 4 in (193 cm) and was looking forward to playing college basketball.

Analysis

Puberty is a time when all adolescents are very conscious of the changes in their bodies and are quick to compare themselves to others. Pete was concerned when he saw boys his age growing taller and developing a masculine physique while he gained height very slowly and experienced few other changes in his appearance. His distress was increased by his commitment to basketball where a player's height is a major factor.

Puberty in boys begins on average between ages 11 and 12, but it can start at any time between ages 9 and 15 and still be considered normal. Puberty begins when the hypothalamus increases the amount of growth hormone-releasing hormone (GHRH) it secretes. It is not clear what triggers this change. Increased GHRH causes the anterior pituitary to double its GH production. The increase in GH is primarily responsible for a rapid gain in height. On average, during puberty, boys gain 3 in (7.6 cm) each year for several years. Before puberty is complete, many boys will have grown 15 in (38 cm) or more.

Increased testosterone production that accompanies male puberty is responsible for maturation of the reproductive organs. It also drives changes in body shape, making the body more muscular and creating the wide shoulders and narrow waist that are characteristic of adult men. Increased body odor and sweating, along with the development of facial and body hair and often severe acne, are also stimulated by increased testosterone.

It would have been better if Pete and his dad had talked to Pete's doctor sooner rather than trying to jump-start Pete's growth with an Internet GH supplement. In the United States, GH is a controlled substance and is recognized as a prohibited performance-enhancing substance by the World Anti-Doping Agency. GH can be used legally only under the direct supervision of a doctor and then only to treat relatively rare and documented medical growth problems.

To get around the question of GH legality, many products are advertised as containing growth hormone releasers that will stimulate the body to naturally increase GH production. Other products claim to contain ingredients that the body will convert into GH. Neither of these statements is true. GH products are considered dietary supplements. They are not regulated by the FDA and may contain impurities and ingredients not listed on the label that at best, will be ineffective and at worst, can be harmful. The only way to get effective GH into the body is by daily injections; pills, gels, and skin creams are worthless, as Pete and his dad found out.

Pete's puberty started late, but starting puberty late does not change the individual's final adult height. Late starters simply grow faster and gain more inches in a shorter amount of time. About 80% of a person's final height is determined by genetics, while the remainder is affected by nutrition and environmental factors. Since Pete's dad was well over six feet,

Pete was likely to end up taller than average, assuming that his mother was of at least normal height.

2. JERRY UNDERGOES GENDER AFFIRMING TREATMENT

Jerry, normally a good student, almost failed two classes during his junior year in high school and was removed from the track team because of alcohol use. When summer came, he refused to look for a job, staying up late and disappearing into his room for hours without explanation. He was obviously unhappy but refused to talk to his parents. They finally convinced him to see a therapist. The therapist recommended that he see a psychiatrist who prescribed medication for Jerry's depression. Jerry's behavior did not change, and when classes began again, he started skipping school.

After months of sessions with the psychiatrist and refusal to talk to his parents, Jerry asked for a family meeting to discuss something he was working through with the psychiatrist.

"This is going to upset you," Jerry told his parents and sister, Emma. "I've always felt I wasn't like other guys. Inside I feel like I am female. I identify with girl's emotions and interests and their way of looking at the world."

"You're telling us you're gay?" his mother asked.

"No," Jerry said. "I'm telling you my internal gender identity and my external appearance don't match. I identify as female. I always have. But I look male. It took a lot of therapy to start to deal with that. My psychiatrist has helped me accept that I have gender dysphoria. I've thought a lot about it, and I want to transition to a female. I need my body to match the way I see myself, and I need the world to see me as female. From now on I want to be called Lucy and use the pronouns she and her."

The family was stunned and distressed. Jerry's father cursed the psychiatrist. He could barely face the idea of losing his only son. His mother cried and prayed and blamed herself. Emma spent as much time out of the house as she could.

After learning more about gender dysphoria, the family made the difficult adjustment to the idea that Lucy was serious. At Lucy's request, the family attended education and therapy sessions with a psychiatrist who specialized in gender dysphoria. Slowly they came to understand what Lucy needed and what her transition would involve.

At first Lucy wanted to tell the high school that she was transitioning, but after discussions with her psychiatrist and parents, she decided that with high school ending in a few months, she would continue as Jerry in school. The community the family lived in was conservative, and she did not want to fight battles over which bathroom to use or have to explain her transition to people she probably would never see again. She even worried about getting beaten up.

Once classes ended, Lucy let her hair grow long and began taking hormones that would remodel her body into a more feminine shape. She did try to explain her gender transformation to her closest friends. Her announcement was met with everything from complete rejection to questions and attempts at understanding. She looked forward to starting college where everyone would know her only as Lucy.

The college Lucy attended was in a city where she could continue to work with a psychiatrist and a doctor who specialized in treating trans people. She progressed with hormone therapy and was happy with her developing breasts. When she went home for winter break, her feminine body was starting to be obvious. While at home, she happened to meet one of Emma's friends downtown.

"What's wrong with your brother?" the friend later asked Emma. "He looks different."

"Nothing's wrong with him," Emma said. "That's my sister, Lucy."

"What do you mean?"

Emma hated these conversations, but she was a loyal sister. "Jerry has transitioned and is Lucy. Inside she always felt like she was female—almost like she was born with the wrong body—and it made her unhappy. She wants to present herself to the world in the same way that she sees herself. She changed her name and her pronouns and is taking hormones to make her body feminine."

"Eww," said the friend. "That's weird. Is she going to have surgery to—you know—get female body parts?"

"That's up to her," Emma snapped. "It really is no one else's business. Right now, she just wants to be accepted for who she is."

Analysis

Jerry was experiencing gender dysphoria, the feeling that his internal gender identity and his assigned sex at birth did not match. This caused him a huge amount of stress that resulted in depression and acting out. Fortunately, Lucy found a psychiatrist who could treat her depression and help her sort through her feelings to come to an understanding about her identity.

Families often find it difficult to understand why their child needs to transition. Many reject the idea completely. They may feel their child's transition reflects badly on them, blame themselves, believe transition is against their religious faith, or refuse to admit gender dysphoria is real. Lucy's decision to transition was not made lightly, and she was fortunate that her parents and sister, although struggling with the change, were willing to learn and support her.

Although announcing a change in one's name and pronouns usually is the first step to transitioning, hormone therapy is what creates changes in body shape. The process takes several years. Lucy needed to understand the risks and benefits of hormone therapy before she began this phase of transition. Common risks include developing blood clots, an increased risk of stroke, high blood pressure, high cholesterol, liver disease, an increased chance of developing type 2 diabetes, and loss of fertility. Hormones are not suitable for everyone, and their use must be supervised by a physician experienced in transition medicine. The process often stimulates a roller coaster of emotional changes, including worsening anxiety and depression for which Lucy was treated. Some physical changes brought about by her hormone treatment would be permanent.

Lucy began by taking testosterone blockers. These suppress her male reproductive functions and over time reduce the size of her testicles. Meanwhile, she began taking estrogens to acquire a female shape. Estrogens caused her skin to thin, reduced her facial and body hair, and gradually changed her body shape so that the amount of fat around her hips and thighs increased. In addition, she lost muscle mass and strength so that her body contour was softened.

As estrogen therapy progressed, breast buds developed under Lucy's nipples. With continuing estrogen therapy, these will develop into breasts, just as they do in a young girl who goes through puberty. Meanwhile, Lucy continued seeing a therapist. People who work with a therapist throughout their transition have been shown to be happier with their transition.

3. MARIE IS SERIOUS ABOUT DANCE

Fifteen-year-old Marie started taking ballet when she was three. She loved the discipline of dance and worked hard to build her skills. Her work had paid off when she earned a place in a nationally recognized ballet school. One day the ballet master looked at the girls working at the barre and said, "Marie, you look like you've gained a few pounds. Remember there's no place here for a pudgy dancer."

Marie was crushed by her teacher's harsh words. The girls in the program constantly talked about what they weighed and what they did and didn't eat. Although she had never had trouble keeping her weight down,

Marie began to diet rigorously. It did not help that one of the mean, competitive girls started calling her Pudge.

Over the next six months, Marie lost weight. Every time she was hungry, she remembered the ballet master's words. She felt exhausted much of the time, and the pleasure she got from dancing began slipping away. Soon her menstrual periods became sporadic. One day she realized she had not menstruated in three months. She knew she could not be pregnant, but after another month without a period, she was worried enough to see a doctor.

The doctor examined Marie and asked about her menstrual history, sleep habits, and demands of the ballet program. She also confirmed that Marie was not pregnant. When asked about her diet, Marie exaggerated a bit about how much she ate. She didn't want the doctor to bring up eating disorders, something dancers were frequently cautioned about.

"You are in a very competitive program, and it could be stress that is causing your missed periods," the doctor said. "But four months is a long time at your age not to menstruate. You are also underweight. Your body mass index is 17.3. Anything under 18.5 is considered underweight, so that is likely contributing to your failure to menstruate. We'll do some tests and see what shows up."

A few days later, the test results came in. Most of the readings were at the low end of the normal range, but Marie's thyroid hormones and estrogen level were seriously below normal, and her cortisol was high. The doctor requested some additional tests for confirmation and then spoke to Marie again.

"Your stress hormones are about double what is considered normal," the doctor said. "And you are substantially undernourished. That combination is likely why you have stopped menstruating. Your thyroid hormones are also low, which contributes to your exhaustion. I don't believe you have an eating disorder yet, but you are headed in that direction, and that is one place you do not want to go."

"But I can't afford to gain weight," Marie said. "Not if I want to succeed in ballet."

"You can't afford *not* to eat more, or you will become seriously sick," the doctor said. "I am referring you to a nutritionist who can help you develop a realistic diet. I understand your concerns as a dancer, but you need to maintain your health. If you keep on the path, you have started down, you can do permanent damage to your body. Pretty soon your bones will start to weaken and eventually there is a good chance that you will break something and not be able to dance at all."

Marie saw the nutritionists and reluctantly took some of her advice. She had seen other dancers starve themselves or throw up in the bathroom after eating what they thought was too much food. She didn't want to be like them, but her fear of gaining weight was strong. Slowly, she gained a few pounds and felt more energetic and happier with herself. Her periods returned but remained irregular. She stayed in the training program, and the ballet master did not mention the few pounds she had gained.

Analysis

A few thoughtless words can send a dancer like Marie, an ice skater, jockey, model, or anyone who needs to stay at a low weight to succeed in their chosen field into a tailspin of dieting that can eventually lead to an eating disorder. Starvation, whether self-imposed or due to a lack of available food, sets the body on a quest to reduce energy use. This is reflected in changes in hormone production.

In Marie's case, the doctor identified three major hormones that were abnormal. The first change Marie noticed was that her menstrual periods had stopped. When the body is starved, the hypothalamus reduces and then stops releasing gonadotropin-releasing hormone (GnRH). This begins a cascade of reactions. Without GnRH, the anterior pituitary does not produce follicle-stimulating hormone (FSH) or luteinizing hormone (LH). In the absence of these hormones, Marie's ovaries failed to produce enough estrogen for an egg to mature. Even if an egg did mature, the lack of LH would prevent it from bursting out of its follicle and entering the fallopian tubes where fertilization could occur (see question 15).

Although Marie was not sexually active, if she were, she would be highly unlikely to conceive a child. Pregnancy puts high demands on the body's energy stores. When food is not available, making conception difficult is one way for the body to protect itself from any excess energy demands.

Marie also had low concentrations of thyroid hormones. Thyroid hormones regulate metabolism, or the speed at which the body uses energy. In times of starvation, the hypothalamus reduces the amount of thyroid-releasing hormone (TRH) it produces. This, in turn, reduces the amount of thyroid-stimulating hormone (TSH) secreted by the anterior pituitary. The result is that the thyroid produces fewer hormones, and body metabolism slows. By slowing metabolism, the body once again is conserving its energy resources. The result was that Marie often felt exhausted, depressed, and unusually sensitive to cold.

Cortisol is a hormone released by the adrenal cortex when the body is under stress. Studies have shown that people with eating disorders have on average double the normal concentration of cortisol. In Marie's case, stress could have come from the demands of her training program, her rigorous dieting, or both. In any case, cortisol causes a rise in blood pressure, a decrease in thyroid hormones, anxiety, depression, and sleep problems.

The doctor also mentioned that over time, Marie's bones might soften and weaken. This can be a long-term result of too little calcium in the diet. To compensate, parathyroid hormone (PTH) increases. This causes calcium to be dissolved out of bones. Over time, bones can become weaker and more susceptible to breaking, something commonly seen in the elderly. Although there is only a small chance that this would happen to Marie, the doctor wanted to impress on her the potential consequences of her starvation diet.

Fortunately, Marie was wise enough to go to the doctor and to reluctantly follow the nutritionist's advice, even though she continued to be concerned about gaining weight. Over time, she learned to recognize her body's needs and how to balance them with the physical requirements of ballet.

4. ANTHONY HAS HASHIMOTO THYROIDITIS

"Are you coming with me to the gym?" asked Jessica, Anthony's wife.

"Nah, not today." Anthony stretched out on the couch and reached for the TV remote. "I'm exhausted."

"You say that almost every time I suggest we get some exercise." Jessica tossed workout clothes into her gym bag. "You complain that you've gained 15 pounds, but when I want us to go to the gym or out for a run, you're always too tired. What's your problem? You used to like to exercise."

"You go," Anthony said. "I told you, I'm beat. And before you leave, can you turn up the heat? It's freezing in here."

"Feels okay to me," Jessica said. But she flipped the thermostat up a couple of degrees before she left.

When the couple married 13 years ago, Anthony had been a lean, well-muscled gym rat who never passed up the opportunity to work out. In fact, it was Anthony who had gotten Jessica started on a fitness routine. But now, despite her prodding and encouragement, all Anthony wanted to do when he got home work was sit on the couch and play video games. Mostly he complained that he was tired. Sometimes he complained that his muscles ached, even though he had done nothing more physical than load the dishwasher.

When Jessica returned from the gym, Anthony was asleep on the couch. She took a good look at her sleeping husband. His face was puffy, his skin pale and dry, and his hair thin and brittle. The changes had come on so slowly that she hadn't really registered them until now. Something, she decided, was definitely wrong. Later that night, she brought up the subject of Anthony's exhaustion.

"You just aren't yourself," she said and listed the things about Anthony that had changed. "Maybe you're depressed. What about seeing a therapist?"

"I'm not depressed," Anthony snapped. "I'm just tired."

"You're always tired. That's not normal. It's not like you work construction. You've got a desk job. If you don't want to see a therapist, maybe you should see the doctor. You haven't had a checkup in years."

"Nag, nag, nag," said Anthony. And he went to bed.

Anthony continued to drag himself through his days, and Jessica continued to remind him that his level of exhaustion was not normal.

"Anthony," Jessica said one night after another grumble about his lack of energy. "If you go get a physical and the doctor says everything is okay, I'll stop bugging you. Okay?"

Anthony grudgingly agreed to schedule a physical. The initial routine blood work showed that his thyroid-stimulating hormone (TSH) produced by the anterior pituitary was abnormally high, but his level of thyroid hormone was abnormally low. The doctor ordered some follow-up tests and a more extensive examination. When all the results were in, the doctor told Anthony he appeared to have Hashimoto thyroiditis and referred him to an endocrinologist who confirmed the diagnosis.

"Don't worry," the endocrinologist said. "This is completely treatable with thyroid hormone supplements. We'll figure out the right dose, and you'll take a daily pill, but you'll have to do this for the rest of your life."

Anthony took the thyroid hormone pills. Within a few weeks, he began to feel more energetic. Within three months, many of his other symptoms had almost disappeared, and he was back doing light workouts in the gym.

Analysis

Hashimoto thyroiditis is an autoimmune disease of the thyroid. It is the most common cause of hypothyroidism in the United States. Each year it is diagnosed in about 4 of every 1,000 women and in 1 of every 1,000 men. Initially, symptoms are general and often are attributed to other causes, so the actual rates are likely higher. The disorder can run in families, but it can also develop spontaneously.

For some unknown reason, Anthony's immune system had targeted and killed many of his thyroid cells. Although his healthy anterior pituitary produced adequate TSH, his thyroid was under attack from his misguided immune system. When enough thyroid cells had been killed, it became impossible for the gland to produce an adequate amount of thyroid hormones. The hypothalamus, or master regulator of metabolism, registered that inadequate thyroid hormones were circulating in the blood. Because the level was low, it signaled the anterior pituitary to produce more TSH, but the thyroid remained unable to respond. This failure disrupted the normal feedback loop that regulates the level of thyroid hormone in the blood and explains why blood tests showed that Anthony's TSH level was extremely high, but his thyroid hormone levels were low.

Thyroid hormones help regulate basic body metabolism. This includes body temperature, heart rate, breathing rate, rate of digestion, body weight, sperm maturation in men and menstrual cycles in women, muscle strength, cholesterol level, and sleep quality. Anthony had some classic signs of hypothyroidism: sensitivity to cold; unexplained weight gain; puffy face; pale skin; and brittle, thinning hair. Because these symptoms developed gradually, he ignored them. The fact that Anthony had so many distinctive symptoms suggests that he had had a thyroid deficiency for months or years.

After his physical, Anthony was referred to an endocrinologist who ruled out the possibility of thyroid cancer or other causes of thyroid hormone deficiency. Once the correct replacement dose of thyroid hormone was determined, Anthony started on supplement pills. The pills are very safe but must be taken for the remainder of his life.

5. LUCIA'S HORMONES CREATE AN ATHLETIC CONFLICT

Lucia, a middle-distance runner, is a world-class track-and-field athlete. Her specialty is 800 meters. She competes regularly in high-visibility international events, including past Olympics, where she won her event. One day, in 2018, Lucia's coach appeared looking serious.

"I have some very upsetting news," he said. "It's going to affect whether you can continue to compete."

"What?" Lucia said. "I'm training really well. I feel great, and you know I follow the rules and don't mess with drugs."

"I know, but you have a very high level of testosterone," the coach said. "Today the International Association of Athletics Federations (IAAF) released new regulations that say any woman whose testosterone level is above five nanomoles per liter must either take hormones to reduce her testosterone or compete against men."

"My testosterone is way above that," Lucia said. "That's just the way my body works. You know I don't take testosterone supplements or use steroids. I never have."

The coach shook his head. He knew Lucia was telling the truth. Her body simply made a lot of testosterone—more than any woman he had ever coached—and he knew she had never used performance-enhancing drugs.

"Apparently a well-known medical journal published a study that showed excessive levels of testosterone in women give them an unfair advantage over women with what are considered 'normal' female testosterone levels. World Athletics is going to enforce the new IAAF testosterone rule for track-and-field athletes starting in a couple of months. They say this will create a level playing field for all women. To continue to compete, you have to take female hormones that will bring your testosterone level down. This ruling will affect track-and-field athletes like you and possibly trans male-to-female athletes."

"What are we going to do?" Lucia asked. "I don't want to take hormones to change my body. I want to compete as me in the body I was born with."

"We can fight this in court as discrimination," said the coach, "but it will be slow going, and you may have passed your performance peak before the court reaches a decision."

Lucia started to cry. "I'm a woman. I've always been a woman. I've worked so hard for so long. Why can't I just run as myself?" she sobbed.

Analysis

Lucia naturally makes levels of testosterone that are much higher than those found in most women. In fact, they are much closer to the level that some male athletes make. This occurs because she has a rare genetic disorder of sexual differentiation (DSD). Her chromosomes are XY, which usually indicate a male, rather than XX, the female pattern. When Lucia was born, her genitals were not fully female, but they were definitely not male. She was assigned female at birth by the doctor and her family. Her gender identity—that deeply held sense of self and what gender she is—had always been female, and her sexual orientation was strictly heterosexual.

During the first six weeks of pregnancy, all fetuses contain tissue that can become either male or female sex organs. In the presence of androgens, fetuses develop male sex organs. When androgens are absent, fetuses develop as females. Estrogens do not have to be present for this to happen;

the absence of androgens is enough to create female sex organs and to suppress male ones.

Normally, androgens are present in early pregnancy in XY fetuses and absent in XX fetuses, so chromosomal sex and the individual's sex organs match. However, between 1 in 20,000 and 1 in 64,000 XY fetuses are born with a condition called androgen insensitivity. Androgens are present in the fetal body, but the tissue that is supposed to differentiate into male sex organs does not respond or responds very minimally to them. The lack of response to androgens causes the fetus to develop primarily female sex organs despite having XY (male) chromosomes. Later, the Y chromosome directs other parts of the body such as the adrenal glands to make excess androgens, a condition known as hyperandrogenism. The result is a person who appears physically female, has female gender identity, and who has levels of testosterone close to male levels. This is important in many sports because testosterone generally increases muscle mass, muscle strength, and the number of oxygen-carrying red blood cells, all conditions that can give an advantage to an athlete.

The IAAF and World Athletics, the governing body for track and field, found that 7 of every 1,000 elite female track-and-field athletes have excessively high testosterone levels. This finding, along with research showing testosterone can improve physical performance, caused these organizations to create a limit on the blood level of testosterone that people competing as females could have. The organizations argued that high testosterone gave these women an unfair advantage over other female competitors. To continue to compete, women with high testosterone would have to take hormones to reduce their natural levels of testosterone to "normal" female levels, or they could choose to compete against men. The women with hyperandrogenism claimed that they were being discriminated against.

Athletic organizations in sports where athletes compete only against individuals of their own apparent sex are grappling with how to handle what they call "intersex" individuals like Lucia as well as people who have undergone gender transformation to become physically the opposite gender while having nonconforming sex chromosomes. These situations create the challenge of providing a level playing field for all competitors while avoiding discrimination on the basis of gender and/or a genetic "disability."

Some banned track-and-field athletes have already appealed the testosterone ruling to the Court of Arbitration for Sports. It ruled against the athletes and for World Athletics. Some scientists now claim that the study that led to the new rules failed to show cause and effect and was inadequate for making such a sweeping ruling. As of late 2021, a case like Lucia's had been brought before the European Court of Human Rights, which at the time this book was written had not yet made a ruling. Meanwhile, World Athletics has agreed that more studies of the relationship between high testosterone and female athletic performance should be done, but they continue to enforce the rule that prevents women with unmodified hyperandrogenism from competing internationally.

❖❖❖

Directory of Resources

BOOKS

Epstein, Randi Hutter. *Aroused*. New York: Norton, 2018.
Fifteen stories about the discovery and function of hormones from the 1850s to the 2020s.
Luck, Martin. *Hormones: A Very Short Introduction*. Oxford, UK: Oxford University Press, 2014.
Compact description of hormone functions for adult readers.
Scott, Celicia. *Doping: Human Growth Hormone, Steroids, & Other Performance-Enhancing Drugs*. Broomall, PA: Mason Crest, 2015.
Basic information for younger readers.

ORGANIZATIONS

American College of Obstetricians and Gynecologists
PO Box 96920
Washington, DC 20024
https://www.acog.org
Professional physicians' organization providing patient information about all aspects of women's reproductive health, including FAQs for teens.

American Diabetes Association
2541 Crystal Drive, Suite 900

Alexandria, VA 22202
1-800-DIABETES (1-800-342-2383)
https://www.diabetes.org
Extensive information about type 1 and type 2 diabetes, including current treatments and research advances.

British Thyroid Foundation
Suite 12, One Sceptre House
Hornbeam Square North
Hornbeam Park
Harrogate
HG2 8PB
+44 (0)1423 810093
info@btf-thyroid.org
An organization providing extensive information about thyroid diseases and current research.

Endocrine Society
2055 L Street NW, Suite 600
Washington, DC 20036
202-971-3636
https://www.endocrine.org
A professional organization for advancing hormone research and improving the clinical practice of endocrinology.

Human Growth Foundation
997 Glen Cove Ave, Suite 5
Glen Head, New York 11545 USA
800-451-6434 toll-free
516-671-4055 fax
hgf1@hgfound.org
https://www.hgfound.org
An organization involved in endocrine research, education, patient advocacy, and public awareness of individuals with growth disorders.

MAGIC Foundation
4200 Cantera Dr. #106
Warrenville, IL 60555
800-362-4423 toll-free
630-836-8181 fax
contact@magicfoundation.org

https://www.magicfoundation.org
An organization devoted to people with growth hormone disorders.

Office of Women's Health
U.S. Department of Health and Human Services
200 Independence Avenue, S.W.
Washington, DC 20201
800-994-9662 toll-free
https://www.womenshealth.gov
A federal government website that provides women's health information in 16 different languages.

Pituitary Foundation
86 Colston Street, Bristol, BS1 5BB, UK
+44 117 370 1333
+44 117 933 0910
enquiries@pituitary.org.uk
https://www.pituitary.org.uk
A UK organization with an extensive website specializing in pituitary disorders.

Planned Parenthood Federation of America
PO Box 97166
Washington, DC 20090-7166
800-430-4907
https://www.plannedparenthood.org
Information online on all aspects of reproduction and in-person services at many local offices.

Society for Endocrinology
Starling House
1600 Bristol Parkway North
Bristol
BS34 8YU
United Kingdom
https://www.endocrinology.org
A professional UK organization with information for students and patients.

Society of Obstetricians and Gynaecologists of Canada
2781 Lancaster Road, Suite 200

Ottawa, ON K1B 1A7
613-730-4192 or 1-800-561-2416
https://sogc.org
Canadian physicians' organization providing patient information about
all aspects of women's reproductive health in English and French.

VIDEOS

All about Boys Puberty. Wellcast. April 12, 2014. https://www.youtube.com
/watch?v=uDmTeU6H40s
An animated video describing the changes boys go through in puberty.

Bone Homeostasis (Calcium and Phosphate) Hormones. Hasudungan, Armando.
February 26, 2012. https://www.youtube.com/watch?v=qDmjNtf5VsE
A podcast on hormones affecting bones with drawings and diagrams of
their actions.

The Fantastical World of Hormones with Dr John Wass. Spark. February 27,
2018. https://www.youtube.com/watch?v=EHnJjGzp__M
A documentary on the discovery of hormones.

The Hypothalamus and Pituitary Gland. Khan Academy. September 18,
2013. https://www.youtube.com/watch?v=9dS7bc_2bUE
An explanation of the relationship of the hypothalamus and pituitary in
endocrine control.

Hypothalamic Pituitary Thyroid Axis (Regulation, TRH, TSH, Thyroid Hormones T3 and T4). Hasudungan, Armando. June 24, 2019. https://www
.youtube.com/watch?v=KzM8BiSnKQM
An explanation of how thyroid hormones are regulated.

Stress Response Physiology. Bhattacharjee, Suman. November 16, 2016.
https://www.youtube.com/watch?v=sWZWjPob0hQ
An explanation of the actions of stress hormones.

What Is Puberty? Decoding Puberty in Girls Wellcast. April 13, 2014.
https://www.youtube.com/watch?v=Tr8ZSH3eghs
An animated video describing the changes girls go through in puberty.

WEBSITES

Biology Libre Texts
"Hormones"

https://bio.libretexts.org
A free U.S. Department of Education textbook project from the University of California, Davis.
Hormone Health Network
https://www.hormone.org
An online resource from the Endocrine Society providing information in many languages on hormones and their effects on health.

Human Rights Campaign Resources on Gender-Expansive Children and Youth
https://www.hrc.org/resources/resources-on-gender-expansive
-children-and-youth
An extensive list of support groups and literature for parents, educators, and young people concerning nontraditional sexual identity.

Merck Manual Professional Version. Female Reproductive Endocrinology.
https://www.merckmanuals.com/professional/gynecology-and
-obstetrics/female-reproductive-endocrinology/female-reproductive
-endocrinology
A detailed review of both the physical and hormonal changes that occur from puberty through menopause.

Pathophysiology of the Endocrine System
Fundamental Concepts in Endocrinology
http://www.vivo.colostate.edu/hbooks/pathphys/endocrine/index.html
A basic tour of the endocrine system developed by Colorado State University.

You and Your Hormones
https://www.yourhormones.info
An online resource from the Society for Endocrinology providing information for students and classroom activities for teachers.

Glossary

Adrenal: A small gland located at the top of each kidney.

Adrenal cortex: The outer part of the adrenal gland that produces the hormones cortisol, aldosterone, and dehydroepiandrosterone (DHEA).

Adrenal medulla: The inner part of the adrenal gland that produces "fight or flight" hormones epinephrine and norepinephrine to prepare the body for action.

Adrenocorticotropic hormone (ACTH): A hormone released by the anterior pituitary that causes the adrenal cortex to produce cortisol.

Aldosterone: A hormone produced by the adrenal cortex that helps to regulate fluid balance and blood pressure by affecting the chemical content of urine removed from the body.

Alpha cell: A type of cell in the pancreas that produces the hormone glucagon when blood glucose levels fall below normal.

Amenorrhea: The absence of menstrual periods for three or more months after regular menstrual cycles have been established.

Anabolic: A substance that increases protein synthesis and builds up tissues in the body.

Antidiuretic hormone (ADH): Also called vasopressin. A hormone made in the hypothalamus and released by the posterior pituitary. It regulates the amount of urine made by the kidneys.

Beta cells: Cells in the pancreas that secrete insulin into the bloodstream when blood glucose levels rise above normal.

Bioaccumulate: The way some harmful chemicals become concentrated in the body instead of being flushed out in waste products or converted into other chemicals that the body can use.

Body mass index (BMI): A weight-to-height ratio used to define the conditions of being underweight, normal weight, overweight, or obese.

Calcitonin: A hormone made by endocrine cells embedded in, but independent of, the thyroid gland that helps regulate calcium balance by activating osteoblast cells to produce new bone.

Corpus luteum: A body formed from the remains of an ovarian follicle that has released a mature egg. It produces progesterone to prepare the uterus for implantation.

Corticotropin-releasing hormone (CRH): A hormone made in the hypothalamus that stimulates the anterior pituitary to secrete adreno-corticotropic hormone.

Cortisol: A hormone produced by the adrenal cortex that affects blood pressure and helps suppress inflammation. It is sometimes called the stress hormone.

Dehydroepiandrosterone (DHEA): A hormone produced by the adrenal cortex that is converted into testosterone in males and estrogen in females.

Electrolytes: Salts and minerals that ionize in body fluids. Electrolytes control fluid balance and are important in muscle contraction, energy generation, and almost all biochemical reactions.

Endocrine disruptors: Chemicals that block the normal action of hormones.

Endometrium: The lining of the uterus.

Epinephrine: Also called adrenaline. A short-acting stress hormone that increases heart rate so that more blood goes to muscles and the brain in preparation for fight or flight.

Estrogen: Also spelled oestrogen. The most common way of referring to a group of the three feminizing hormones: estradiol, estriol, and estrone.

Exocrine cells: Cells that secrete their products into a duct to be transported as opposed to endocrine cells that secrete their products directly into the bloodstream.

Fallopian tube: A tube adjacent to each ovary that transports an egg to the uterus. Fertilization of the egg occurs in the fallopian tube.

Follicle: The thin sack of cells surrounding a developing egg in the ovary that bursts when the egg is mature so that fertilization can occur.

Follicle-stimulating hormone (FSH): Both men and women make this hormone under stimulation of gonadotropin-releasing hormone. It affects the maturation and function of both male and female reproductive organs.

Gender dysphoria: The condition of having one's strong internal sense of gender in conflict with one's biological sex assigned at birth.

Gender identity: A deeply held sense of maleness, femaleness, or identification with both genders that is independent of assigned biological sex or sexual orientation.

Glucagon: A hormone secreted by alpha cells in the pancreas that signals the liver to break down glycogen into glucose and release it into the bloodstream when blood glucose levels are too low.

Gonadotropin-releasing hormone (GnRH): A hormone secreted by the hypothalamus that stimulates the release of follicle-stimulating hormone and luteinizing hormone in both males and females.

Growth hormone (GH): A hormone secreted by the anterior pituitary under stimulation by growth hormone-releasing hormone from the hypothalamus. It moderates growth and increases substantially during puberty.

Gynecomastia: The enlargement of breast tissue in men. This is common in boys going through puberty and will normally resolve without treatment.

Homeostasis: Body conditions such as temperature, fluid balance, or blood chemistry that must be maintained within a narrow range for the body to remain healthy.

Hydrophilic: Literally, water loving. A substance that can dissolve in water.

Hypothalamus: A region of the brain that serves as the connection between the nervous and endocrine systems. It monitors blood chemistry and secretes releasing hormones that stimulate the pituitary.

Insulin: A hormone produced by beta cells in the pancreas that decreases the amount of glucose in the blood.

Lipophilic: Literally, fat loving. A substance that can dissolve in fat or oil.

Luteinizing hormone (LH): A hormone produced by the anterior pituitary under stimulation by gonadotropin-releasing hormone made in the hypothalamus. In women LH causes the release of a mature egg from a follicle. In men it stimulates the testes to produce testosterone.

Melatonin: A hormone made in the pineal gland that helps to regulate the sleep-wake cycle.

Menarche: The time of a girl's first menstrual period, most often between ages 12 and 13.

Menopause: The time when a woman's menstrual period stops and she can no longer conceive a child, usually between ages 45 and 55.

Metabolism: The chemical reactions in every cell that turn nutrients into energy for the body.

Neurotransmitter: Any of a group of chemicals released by a nerve cell that allows the nerve impulse to cross the space between nerve cells so that transmission of the nerve impulse is not interrupted.

Nonbinary: An individual who self-identifies as neither strictly male nor strictly female.

Norepinephrine: Also called noradrenaline: A short-acting hormone produced by the adrenal medulla under conditions of fear and stress. It helps increase focus and supplements the actions of epinephrine in preparing the body for action. In non-stressful situations, it is secreted by nerve endings and can affect mood.

Oligomenorrhea: Infrequent menstrual periods, usually less than six to eight per year.

Osteoblasts: Cells that are activated by the presence of the hormone calcitonin to build up new bone and remove calcium from the blood.

Osteoclasts: Cells that, when activated by the release of parathyroid hormone, break down old bone so that calcium ions are released and the concentration of calcium in the blood rises.

Oxytocin: A hormone made by the hypothalamus and stored in the pituitary until it is released. It stimulates contractions during childbirth and social bonding. Men also make oxytocin. Its purpose in men is unclear but is thought to relate to social behavior.

Pancreas: A gland located behind the stomach on the left side of the body that produces two main hormones, insulin and glucagon.

Parathyroid: Four tiny glands in the neck behind the thyroid that produce parathyroid hormone, which regulates the amount of calcium in the blood.

Parathyroid hormone (PTH): Hormone produced by the parathyroid gland whose only purpose is to regulate the amount of calcium in the blood.

Pineal: A gland located deep within the brain that produces the hormone melatonin in response to the amount of light entering the eye.

Pituitary: A gland closely associated with the hypothalamus. It is divided into an anterior and posterior portion. The anterior pituitary makes six major hormones. The posterior pituitary stores and then releases two hormones made by the hypothalamus.

Primary messenger: A lipophilic (fat loving) hormone that can enter a cell by directly dissolving in the fat that is part of a cell membrane.

Progesterone: A female hormone produced by the corpus luteum and the placenta that is necessary to maintain pregnancy.

Progestin: A synthetic form of progesterone found in oral contraceptives.

Prolactin: A hormone made by the anterior pituitary when stimulated by prolactin-releasing hormone from the hypothalamus. It causes pregnant and nursing women to make breast milk. Men also make prolactin, although scientists do not know why.

Receptor: A structure on the surface or in the interior of the cell that binds only with a specific substance. For example, every cell has a receptor on its surface for insulin.

Releasing hormones: Hormones made by the hypothalamus that direct the production and release of other hormones made by the anterior pituitary.

Secondary messenger: A substance that is generated by a hydrophilic (water loving) hormone when it meets its target cell. The hormone binds with a receptor in the cell membrane. This generates the secondary messenger inside the cell that changes the cell's activities. The hormone itself never enters the cell.

Tanner stages: A description of physical changes in girls and boys during puberty developed by James Tanner to evaluate the progression of puberty independent of chronological age.

Target cell: The cell a hormone acts on to change its activity.

Testosterone: An androgen (male) hormone produced by the testes that stimulates the development of male secondary sexual characteristics and is needed for sperm production, sex drive, and sexual performance. Women also produce a small amount of testosterone.

Thyroid: A gland in the neck that produces two hormones, triiodothyronine (T3) and thyroxine (T4), normally just called thyroid hormones. These help regulate cellular metabolism.

Thyroid-stimulating hormone (TSH): A hormone made by the anterior pituitary under stimulation by thyrotropin-releasing hormone secreted by the hypothalamus. It causes the thyroid gland to make and release thyroid hormones.

Transgender: Individuals whose gender identity does not match the sex they were assigned at birth and who choose to use social, hormonal, and/or surgical means to align their sex with their gender identity.

Bibliography

"Added Sugar in the Diet." Harvard University School of Public Health. n.d https://www.hsph.harvard.edu/nutritionsource/carbohydrates /added-sugar-in-the-diet (accessed September 1, 2021).

"A Dose of Vitamin D History." *Nature Structural Biology* 9, no. 77 (February 2002). https://www.nature.com/articles/nsb0202-77 (accessed July 4, 2020).

Agraharkar, Mahendra. "Hypercalcemia." Medscape. October 3, 2018. https://emedicine.medscape.com/article/240681-overview (accessed July 4, 2020).

Aliyari, Hamad, Hedayat Sahraei, Mohammad Reza Daliri, Behrouz Minaei-Bidgoli, Masoomeh Kazemi, Hassan Agaei, Mohammad Sahraei, et al. "The Beneficial or Harmful Effects of Computer Game Stress on Cognitive Functions of Players." *Basic and Clinical Neuroscience* 9, no. 3 (May–June 2018): 177–186. https://www.ncbi.nlm.nih.gov/pmc /articles/PMC6037427 (accessed September 28, 2021).

Ayyar, Vageesh S. "History of Growth Hormone Therapy." *Indian Journal of Endocrinology and Metabolism* 15, no. suppl. 3 (September 2011): S162–165. https://www.ncbi.nlm.nih.gov/pmc/articles/PMC3183530 (accessed June 18, 2020).

Berenbaum, Sheri A., and Adriene M. Beltz. "How Early Hormones Shape Gender Development." *Current Opinion in Behavioral Science*

7 (February 2016): 53–60. https://www.ncbi.nlm.nih.gov/pmc/articles /PMC4681519 (accessed August 13, 2021).

"Bone Health." Endocrine Society. June 1, 2019. https://www.hormone .org/your-health-and-hormones/bone-health (accessed July 4, 2020).

Bowen, Richard. "Calcitonin." VIVO Pathophysiology. n.d. http://www .vivo.colostate.edu/hbooks/pathphys/endocrine/thyroid/calcitonin .html (accessed July 4, 2020).

Bowen, Richard. "Growth Hormone (Somatotropin)." VIVO Pathophysiology. n.d. http://www.vivo.colostate.edu/hbooks/pathphys/endocrine /hypopit/gh.html (accessed June 17, 2020).

Brunning, Andy. "How Do Pregnancy Tests Work?" Compound Interest. November 9, 2019. https://www.compoundchem.com/2018/11/09 /pregnancy-tests (accessed July 10, 2020).

Chiu, Allyson. "Female Athletes with Naturally High Testosterone Levels Face Hurdles under New IAAF Rules." *Washington Post.* April 27, 2018. https://www.washingtonpost.com/news/morning-mix/wp/2018/04/27 /female-athletes-with-naturally-high-testosterone-levels-face-hurdles -under-new-iaaf-rules (accessed October 5, 2021).

Davidson, Tish. *What You Need to Know about Diabetes.* Santa Barbara, CA: ABC-CLIO, 2020.

"Disorders of Sex Differentiation." Cleveland Clinic. September 23, 2016. https://my.clevelandclinic.org/health/diseases/16324-disorders-of-sex -differentiation (accessed August 13, 2021).

Emmanuel, Mickey, and Brooke R. Bokor. "Tanner Stages." StatPearls. May 13, 2019. https://www.ncbi.nlm.nih.gov/books/NBK470280 (accessed July 28, 2020).

"Endocrine Disruptors." Emory University School of Medicine Department of Pediatrics. 2019. https://factor.niehs.nih.gov/2019/9/feature/3 -feature-lavender/index.htm (accessed May 26, 2020).

Epstein, Randi Hutter. *Aroused.* New York: Norton, 2018.

Farabee, M. J. "The Endocrine System." 2001. https://www2.estrellamoun tain.edu/faculty/farabee/biobk/BioBookENDOCR.html (accessed June 16, 2020).

Farokhnia, Mehdi, Gray R. McDiarmid, Matthew N. Newmeyer, Vikas Munjal, Osama A. Abulseoud, Marilyn A. Huestis, and Lorenzo Leggio. "Effects of Oral, Smoked, and Vaporized Cannabis on Endocrine Pathways Related to Appetite and Metabolism: A Randomized, Double-Blind, Placebo-Controlled, Human Laboratory Study." *Translational Psychiatry* 10, no. 71 (February 2020). https://www.nature.com /articles/s41398-020-0756-3#Abs1 (accessed September 14, 2021).

Fountain, John H., and Sarah L. Lappin. "Physiology, Renin Angiotensin System." StatPearls. July 22, 2021. https://www.ncbi.nlm.nih.gov/books/NBK470410 (accessed August 30, 2021).

Frank, Michelle. "The Neuroscience of Thirst: How Your Brain Tells You to Look for Water." Harvard University Graduate School of Arts and Sciences. September 26, 2019. https://sitn.hms.harvard.edu/flash/2019/neuroscience-thirst-brain-tells-look-water (accessed August 23, 2021).

Grant, Paul. "21st Century Endocrinology." *Clinical Medicine (London)* 9, no. 5 (October 2009): 459–462. https://www.ncbi.nlm.nih.gov/pmc/articles/PMC4953457 (accessed June 11, 2020).

Harvard Medical School. "Testosterone—What It Does and Doesn't Do." Harvard Health Publishing. August 29, 2019. https://www.health.harvard.edu/drugs-and-medications/testosterone--what-it-does-and-doesnt-do (accessed July 13, 2020).

Harvard Men's Health Watch. "Growth Hormone, Athletic Performance, and Aging." Harvard Health Publishing. June 19, 2018. https://www.health.harvard.edu/diseases-and-conditions/growth-hormone-athletic-performance-and-aging (accessed June 22, 2020).

Henderson, John. "Ernest Starling and 'Hormones': An Historical Commentary." *Journal of Endocrinology* 184, no. 1 (2005): 5–10. https://joe.bioscientifica.com/view/journals/joe/184/1/1840005.xml (accessed June 15, 2020).

Hormone Health Network. "Endocrine-Disrupting Chemicals EDCs." Endocrine Society. May 26, 2020. https://www.hormone.org/your-health-and-hormones/endocrine-disrupting-chemicals-edcs (accessed May 26, 2020).

"Human Growth Hormone." Drug Enforcement Administration Office of Diversion Control. September 2019. https://www.deadiversion.usdoj.gov/drug_chem_info/hgh.pdf (accessed June 22, 2020).

Jewell, Tim. "Risk Factors of Having High or Low Estrogen Levels in Males." Healthline. October 22, 2019. https://www.healthline.com/health/estrogen-in-men (accessed June 16, 2020).

Kahn, Maqsood, Alvin Jose, and Sandeep Sharma. "Physiology, Parathyroid Hormone (PTH)." StatPearls. May 29, 2020. https://www.ncbi.nlm.nih.gov/books/NBK499940 (accessed July 4, 2020).

Kalra, Sanjay, Manash P. Baruah, Rakesh Sahay, and Kanishka Sawhney. "The History of Parathyroid Endocrinology." *Indian Journal of Endocrinology and Metabolism* 17, no. 2 (March–April 2013): 320–322. https://www.ncbi.nlm.nih.gov/pmc/articles/PMC3683213 (accessed July 4, 2020).

Klok, M. D., S. Jakobsdottir, and M. L. Drent. "The Role of Leptin and Ghrelin in the Regulation of Food Intake and Body Weight in Humans: A Review." *Obesity Reviews* 8, no. 1 (January 2007): 21–34. https://onlinelibrary.wiley.com/doi/10.1111/j.1467-789X.2006.00270.x (accessed September 14, 2021).

Knudtson, Jennifer. "Female Reproductive Endocrinology." *Merck Manual Professional Version.* March 2019. https://www.merckmanuals.com/professional/gynecology-and-obstetrics/female-reproductive-endocrinology/female-reproductive-endocrinology (accessed August 3, 2020).

Lewis, James L. "Hypocalcemia." *Merck Manual Professional Version.* 2020. https://www.merckmanuals.com/professional/endocrine-and-metabolic-disorders/electrolyte-disorders/hypocalcemia (accessed July 4, 2020).

Lewis, James L. "Overview of Disorders of Calcium Concentration." *Merck Manual Professional Version.* 2020. https://www.merckmanuals.com/professional/endocrine-and-metabolic-disorders/electrolyte-disorders/overview-of-disorders-of-calcium-concentration (accessed July 4, 2020).

Longman, Jeré. "Scientists Correct Study That Restricted Runners." *New York Times.* August 19, 2021. https://www.nytimes.com/2021/08/18/sports/olympics/intersex-athletes-olympics.html (accessed October 5, 2021).

Luck, Martin. *Hormones: A Very Short Introduction.* Oxford, UK: Oxford University Press, 2014.

MacGill, Markus. "Why Do We Need Testosterone?" *Medical News Today.* February 6, 2019. https://www.medicalnewstoday.com/articles/276013 (accessed July 13, 2020).

Manish, Suneja. "Hypocalcemia." Medscape. August 8, 2018. https://emedicine.medscape.com/article/241893-overview (accessed July 4, 2020).

Misra, Madhusmita, and Anne Kilbanski. "Endocrine Consequences of Anorexia Nervosa." *Lancet Diabetes & Endocrinology* 2, no. 7 (July 2014): 581–592. https://www.ncbi.nlm.nih.gov/pmc/articles/PMC4133106 (accessed October 7, 2021).

National Institute of Alcohol Abuse and Alcoholism. "Alcohol Alert no. 26 PH 352." October 1994. https://pubs.niaaa.nih.gov/publications/aa26.htm (accessed September 28, 2021).

National Institute of Environmental Health Sciences. "Endocrine Disruptors." n.d. https://www.niehs.nih.gov/health/topics/agents/endocrine/index.cfm (accessed May 18, 2020).

National Institutes of Health Office of Dietary Supplements. "Calcium." March 26, 2020. https://ods.od.nih.gov/factsheets/Calcium-Health Professional (accessed July 4, 2020).

Olarescu, Nicoleta C., Kavinga Gunawardane, Troels Krarup Hansen, Niels Møller, and Jens Otto Lunde Jørgensen. "Normal Physiology of Growth Hormone in Adults." In *Endotext*. October 16, 2019. https://www.ncbi.nlm.nih.gov/books/NBK279056 (accessed June 17, 2020).

"Parathyroid Glands, High Calcium, and Hyperparathyroidism." Norman Parathyroid Center. 2020. https://www.parathyroid.com (accessed July 4, 2020).

Porter, Anne Marie, and Paula Goolkasian. "Video Games and Stress: How Stress Appraisals and Game Content Affect Cardiovascular and Emotion Outcomes." *Frontiers in Psychology* 10 (May 2019): 967. https://www.ncbi.nlm.nih.gov/pmc/articles/PMC6524699 (accessed September 28, 2021).

Rachdaoui, Nadia, and Dipak K. Sarkar. "Effects of Alcohol on the Endocrine System." *Endocrine Metabolism Clinic of North America* 42, no. 3 (September 2013): 593–615.

Reynolds, Gretchen. "Raging Hormones." *New York Times*. August 20, 2006. https://www.nytimes.com/2006/08/20/sports/playmagazine/20hgh.html (accessed June 22, 2020).

Scott, Celicia. *Doping: Human Growth Hormone, Steroids, & Other Performance-Enhancing Drugs*. Broomall, PA: Mason Crest, 2015.

Schug, Thaddeus T., Anne F. Johnson, Linda S. Birnbaum, Theo Colborn, Louis J. Guillette, Jr., David P. Crews, Terry Collins, et al. "Minireview: Endocrine Disruptors: Past Lessons and Future Directions." *Molecular Endocrinology* 30, no.8 (August 2016): 833–847. https://academic.oup.com/mend/article/30/8/833/2747295 (accessed May 26, 2020).

Schulster, Michael, Aaron M. Bernie, and Ranjith Ramasamy. "The Role of Estradiol in Male Reproductive Function." *Asian Journal of Andrology* 18, no. 3 (May–June 2016): 435–440.

"Study Finds That Melatonin Content of Supplements Varies Widely." American Academy of Sleep Medicine. February 14, 2017. https://aasm.org/study-finds-that-melatonin-content-of-supplements-varies-widely (accessed August 27, 2021).

"Study of U.S. Adults Finds Strong Association Between Higher Sodium Excretion and Higher Blood Pressure and Association Between Higher Potassium Excretion and Lower Blood Pressure." Centers for Disease Control and Prevention. February 28, 2018. https://www.cdc.gov/salt/research_reviews/sodium_potassium_blood_pressure.htm (accessed August 31, 2021).

Tata, Jamshed R. "One Hundred Years of Hormones." *EMBO Reports* 6, no. 6 (June 2005): 490–496. https://www.ncbi.nlm.nih.gov/pmc/articles/PMC1369102 (accessed June 15, 2020).

Toews, Ingrid, Szimonetta Lohner, Daniela Küllenberg de Gaudry, Harriet Sommer, and Joerg Meerpohl. "Association between Intake of Non-Sugar Sweeteners and Health Outcomes: Systematic Review and Meta-Analyses of Randomised and Non-randomised Controlled Trials and Observational Studies." *British Medical Journal* 364 (January 2019): k4718. https://www.bmj.com/content/364/bmj.k4718 (accessed September 18, 2021).

Tyssowski, Kelsey. "Pee Is for Pregnant: The History and Science of Urine-Based Pregnancy Tests." Harvard University Graduate School of Arts and Sciences. August 31, 2018. http://sitn.hms.harvard.edu/flash/2018/pee-pregnant-history-science-urine-based-pregnancy-tests (accessed July 18, 2020).

van den Beld, Annewieke, Jean-Mark Kaufman, M. Carola Zillikens, Steven Lamberts, Josephine Egan, and Aart J. van der Lely. "The Physiology of Endocrine Systems with Ageing." *Lancet Diabetes and Endocrinology* 6, no. 8 (August 2018): 647–658. https://www.ncbi.nlm.nih.gov/pmc/articles/PMC6089223 (accessed August 29, 2021).

"Vitamin D and Calcium." Endocrine Society. June 30, 2018. https://www.hormone.org/your-health-and-hormones/bone-health/vitamin-d-and-calcium (accessed July 4, 2020).

Wakim, Suzanne, and Mandeep Grewal. "Homeostasis and Feedback." Biology Libre Texts. May 24, 2020. https://bio.libretexts.org/Bookshelves/Human_Biology/Book%3A_Human_Biology_(Wakim_and_Grewal)/10%3A_Introduction_to_the_Human_Body/10.7%3A_Homeostasis_and_Feedback (accessed June 15, 2020).

Wass, John. "The Fantastical World of Hormones." *Endocrinologist.* Spring 2015. http://www.endocrinology.org/endocrinologist/pdf-archive (accessed June 15, 2020).

Weaver, Janelle. "Lavender Oil Linked to Early Breast Growth in Girls." National Institute of Environmental Health Sciences Environmental Factor. September 2019. https://factor.niehs.nih.gov/2019/9/feature/3-feature-lavender/index.htm (accessed May 26, 2020).

Index

About the Author

Tish Davidson, AM, is a medical writer specializing in making technical information accessible to a general readership. She is the author of *Vaccines: History, Science, and Issues*, *The Vaccine Debate*, and *What You Need to Know about Diabetes* as well as contributing to *Biology: A Text for High School Students* and *Adolescent Health & Wellness*. Davidson holds membership in the American Society of Journalists and Authors.